MODERN DYSPHAGIA COOKING

Turn family favorites into dysphagia-friendly dishes.

AUTHORS

Laurie Berger, MBA, RD, LD – Paul Haefner –
John Holahan, BS, MBA – Nancy A. Yezzi, RDN, LD

ADDITIONAL CONTRIBUTORS

Liz Fiala

Sarah Holahan

Patti Housley

Karmen Kortie

Jacqueline Larson, MS, RDN

Leslie Levanovic, MS, CCC-SLP

Maureen Leugers, MBA, RDN

Josh Randall

Kay Strand

Wendy West

SPECIAL THANKS TO

Enrich Creative

Garry McMichael

BROUGHT TO YOU BY

◀ Cover Photo: ▽④ Pureed Beef (Steak or Roast) on page 78

Dedications

"For my ALS Angel, Keith, and mother & best friend, Tre Tre."

– Nancy Yezzi, RDN,LD

"For dysphagia patients and their caregivers."

– Wendy West

"To the caregivers caring for my sister-in-law, Jane, who developed dysphagia due to a brain tumor and who is now able to stay safely hydrated and enjoy her favorite foods."

– Patti Housley, Regional Manager — Florida

"To all who will read this, may you never forget the salt, pepper, and a smile."

– Sydney Baer

"To all my fellow Registered Dietitians who provide compassionate care and share their vast nutritional knowledge with those with dysphagia and their loved ones."

– Laurie Berger, RD, LD

"For my mom, Phyllis, a great cook and even better mother."

– Paul Haefner

"This is dedicated to my husband, Jonny Law — a 3x head and neck cancer survivor:

• Who has experienced first-hand the NEED for these recipes.
• Who has been an integral part of the FORMULATION of these recipes.
• Who has been the patient guinea pig, TASTE TESTING these recipes.
• Who has given his honest FEEDBACK on these recipes.
• And most of all, for all of the HUMOR he has freely offered during this process!"

– Karmen Kortie

"This book is dedicated to all the caregivers around the world that work every day to provide the best and safest food for their loved one(s) that struggle with dysphagia."

– John Holahan, President, SimplyThick, LLC

Table of Contents

From the Heart

Eat! Mangia! Bon Appetit! Eating is a joy and a pleasure for most of us. Do you "live to eat" or "eat to live?" For many, eating is something we hold dear and look forward to each day. It's what makes holidays extra special and daily life more interesting — and brings family and friends together. For others, it's simply a function of daily living but necessary, nonetheless.

I do believe we take this GIFT for granted daily with each mouthful of food, and every bite and swallow. When disease affects someone's ability to chew, swallow, or taste, that person suffers both physically and mentally. Whether you are witnessing a loved one's food struggles or are experiencing it first-hand, it can be devastating. This book was prepared by a team of professionals at SimplyThick who care deeply about helping you and your loved one enjoy nourishing meals with greater ease and safety.

I personally watched the intake struggle of my husband, Keith, due to Amyotrophic Lateral Sclerosis (ALS) for several years, and it taught me many lessons. Oh, the lengths we will go to get a loved one nourished; especially as a Registered Dietitian Nutritionist (RDN), as I am, and food is your "business." We are not going to let anyone, let alone a loved one, become malnourished on our watch. We will do everything possible to help our loved ones manage eating difficulties. Realizing that it's ultimately in the patient's hands and power, not yours, is step #1. You can only suggest, support, provide the goods, and encourage them to experiment, try, consume, and sometimes achieve! You will not hit a home run every day, disappointing but true. When you do hit a home run, it is a banner day! Learn to embrace both types of days early on as it will make things flow and minimize frustration for all.

Another matter to reckon with is that the recipes in this book are a guide that, at times, will need to be adjusted to your particular circumstances and abilities. You may need the food softer or firmer, thinner or thicker, more seasoned, etc. It is not always black and white, prescriptive nor absolute. Try to approach the recipes with an open mind and flexibility. A touch of humor never hurts either. Humor was definitely a part of my daily medicine with Keith. We preferred the healthy shot of endorphins that laughter provided while looking at the ugly, green smoothie I made for Keith, all in the name of health and love! "You drink it if it's so good for you, Ms. Dietitian." He would type this out on his iPad and have it spoken back to us with a British accent. That would crack me up and diffuse my product failure in taste and appearance. Remember, we eat with our eyes, and presentation matters, be it a beautiful glass or decorative plate or molding pureed foods to look realistic and appealing.

The patient's individual journey is one we can't fully experience, but your support matters 100%.

Thank goodness for IDDSI: the International Dysphagia Diet Standardisation Initiative, a new way to better assess and test foods and drinks in a dysphagia texture-modified diet. See Chapter 4 for more details. This system can give you peace of mind that you are on the right track to safe swallowing and appropriate diet consistencies. Yet another GIFT! The term "thick" is subjective and can be interpreted differently among individuals. The IDDSI Framework puts all these items in order. And, it gives us benchmarks to reference for safer swallowing and more enjoyable meals.

If you're a patient reading this book, you are a Hero. I applaud you for trying to nourish your body and support your health! If you are a Caregiver, I support you as well and hope you know that your loved one does, too. Don't take things personally. The patient's individual journey is one we can't fully experience, but your support matters 100%. And, they do appreciate you even on the toughest days, even when the words cannot describe it. It's in there, in the heart.

Our team has packed this cookbook with valuable information and resources, and we hope you enjoy them to the fullest. There are many online resources out there as well. I encourage you to peruse the Internet for support groups, dysphagia tools, and innovative products such as SimplyThick® EasyMix™. I can unabashedly say I wish I had this product when Keith was experiencing his dysphagia. It would have meant the world to us and changed his life, as far as safe intake capabilities and pleasurable food and drinks.

We all wish you the best and hope this cookbook assists you in re-establishing your or your loved one's joy of food and drink!

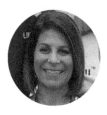

From the Heart —
Nancy Yezzi, RDN, LD

CHAPTER 1

Read This First

WHOA! Slow down and read these few pages FIRST! We know you want to get to cooking, but please pause here for a few moments and "consume" these tips. You will be glad you did.

The recipes in this book are different from traditional recipes. We know that you or your loved one already know how to make the foods you love. Our "recipes" are starting points and training recipes designed to help you learn how to PROCESS your family favorites into food that complies with your prescribed modified diet. Our goal is to help you safely enjoy the foods that have always been on your family's menu as much as possible!

We chose to use the standards of the International Dysphagia Diet Standardisation Initiative (IDDSI). See Chapter 4, which explains IDDSI in more detail. Suffice it to say, IDDSI is revolutionizing the standards of care for dysphagia patients around the globe. The reason is simple: IDDSI gives you three HUGE advantages that will make your texture-modified journey easier:

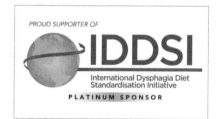

1. Detailed Descriptors of how the food should look, feel, and behave. See Appendix A (p. 184) for reprints of the detailed definitions for Levels 4, 5, and 6. For the most up-to-date version of IDDSI definitions, you can find the "Complete IDDSI Framework Detailed Definitions" document by visiting www.iddsi.org. (This is a remarkable site with many tools and language translations available to help you.)

2. Test Methods that are easy to follow, ensuring that the food has been prepared to perform exactly as the health care professional prescribed it. Serve meals with confidence, knowing that they were prepared to be as safe as possible. See Appendix B (p. 199) for the IDDSI Test Methods. The most up-to-date version of the "IDDSI Framework Testing Methods" document can be found at www.iddsi.org.

3. IDDSI is DESCRIPTIVE. As a global standard, IDDSI has been written to describe food and drink characteristics. There is no authoritative list of acceptable and/or not acceptable foods. If you process the food and

test it and it meets the descriptive standards, you can serve the food. This offers you tremendous flexibility to customize the foods you serve.

The process to modify your food to comply with IDDSI standards is going to be new and different. It is a simple process, but as with anything new, it can feel daunting at first. As you go through the recipes, you will see that the conversion process is fairly straightforward:

1. Prepare food as you normally would.
2. Process the prepared food in a food processor.
3. Evaluate the food using the IDDSI Testing Methods:
   a. Adjust and reprocess in food processor.
   b. Serve and/or store.

Many details go into each step. Once you have learned the tools and the process, we hope you'll become confident in your abilities and use them to explore a variety of different foods!

A Word About Dysphagia

Dysphagia is a swallowing problem: literally pain or difficulty in swallowing. It is a serious medical condition typically diagnosed by a Speech-Language Pathologist (SLP). Do NOT self-diagnose, and do NOT self-treat.

SLPs have deep knowledge of the different food types that can be problematic for persons with dysphagia. Their expertise is invaluable in diagnosing and managing dysphagia. One SLP explained, "Whenever someone describes difficulty eating solids, I typically ask if bread, rice, or lettuce are problematic. The response, usually, is 'Yes,' as people with dysphagia frequently describe difficulty with these three foods due to their size and texture."

Our assumption in writing this book is that you have been to a medical professional — either a doctor, an SLP, or an RDN. We also assume that they have prescribed a specific, textured-modified diet for you or your loved one, and that is the reason you purchased this book: to comply with and follow these medical orders.

If you are not under medical supervision and you are experiencing difficulty or pain when swallowing, please seek medical advice. You may have an undiagnosed medical condition and may benefit from an individualized course of treatment.

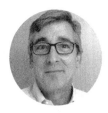

Paul Haefner

CHAPTER 2

Introduction

When I try to explain to friends, family, and new acquaintances what SimplyThick® EasyMix™ is and what dysphagia means, I fall back to this question, "Have you ever had something 'go down the wrong tube' when eating or drinking?"

The answer is always, "Yes, of course." I then follow up with, "If you have a 50/50 chance of every bite of food or sip of a liquid going down the wrong tube, would you go to great lengths — including thickening beverages or modifying meals — to avoid it?" The answer, always, is "Yes, of course."

This cookbook is an extension of our mission to improve the quality of life for individuals with dysphagia. We achieve this by expanding the food and drink options available to them when following a thickened diet, while also making those foods easier to prepare properly, safely, and consistently.

In 2015, the International Dysphagia Diet Standardisation Initiative (IDDSI) was published. The IDDSI Framework provides a common terminology to describe food texture and drink thickness. For those of us who have been working in this field for years, this serves as a game changer in using consistent terms, testing methods, and standards around the world.

The IDDSI Framework aims to standardize the way food is prepared to reduce the risk of choking and aspiration. In doing so, the IDDSI Framework also aims to improve the quality of patients' lives by providing access to a wider variety of safer and healthier diet options. What's most impressive is that these quality-of-life improvements can be achieved anywhere in the world simply by implementing the common practices and terminology that establish the IDDSI Framework.

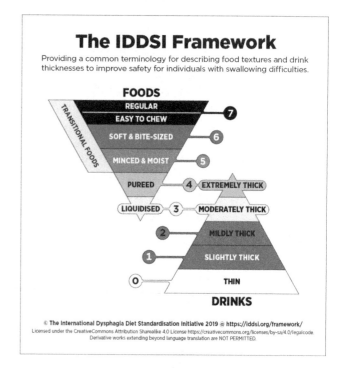

The IDDSI Framework

Providing a common terminology for describing food textures and drink thicknesses to improve safety for individuals with swallowing difficulties.

© The International Dysphagia Diet Standardisation Initiative 2019 @ https://iddsi.org/framework/
Licensed under the CreativeCommons Attribution Sharealike 4.0 License https://creativecommons.org/licenses/by-sa/4.0/legalcode.
Derivative works extending beyond language translation are NOT PERMITTED.

The backbone of the IDDSI Framework is the development of diet levels for adults and children that can be implemented in the same manner across a broad spectrum of care settings.

At typical hospitals, for example, the average length of stay translates to between five and six meals, or two to three days. By the time all of the information and subtleties for a patient can be collected and implemented, that patient is often already on their way home. In hospitals, the food limits (or restrictions) for dysphagia patients are typically hard and fast, even if that means removing a favorite item from the patient's diet.

This cookbook is an extension of our company's mission to improve the quality of life for individuals with dysphagia.

By comparison, in most long-term care facilities the residents and caregivers have months or years together. These situations often permit special 'allowed items' in a resident's Plan of Care once they have been determined to be safe for that resident — even if the item falls outside of a strict interpretation of the prescribed dietary guidelines.

At home, however, the tolerance of a texture modified food item matters only to one person and their medical situation rather than an entire ward of patients. And unlike at a long-term care facility or hospital, at home there isn't the benefit and support of experienced, in-house RDNs and kitchen staff. Typically, a patient is sent home with samples of thickeners and left to their own devices when it comes to food preparation, often while navigating other medical issues at the same time.

IDDSI testing requires ◁4▷ Pureed samples to pass all criteria for 30 minutes after serving the food. Our attempts to puree macaroni and cheese failed because it was 'too sticky' at the 15- and 30-minute markers. We caution all licensed healthcare facilities to avoid macaroni and cheese on ◁4▷ Pureed diets for that reason. You may be at home and make a 4 oz. portion of pureed macaroni and cheese and eat it in less than 7 minutes without complication, choking, or aspirating. You may well be safe. But, if you are subject to pocketing food, aspiration, or spending increased time to consume your meals, the "7 minute mac & cheese" may still pose a specific risk for aspiration. These examples have to be balanced by the overall condition, behavior, and tolerance of a patient. Always consult with your SLP's specific information and instructions for you or your patient.

If you're placed on a ▽6▽ Soft & Bite-Sized menu and enjoy a slice of roast beef with creamy horseradish spread for dinner, you can just cut it into bite-sized pieces and you're ready to eat. But, if the spicy horseradish sauce produces excess saliva that causes loss of control of the food bolus (the medical term for a soft chewed mass of food ready to swallow), or causes you to choke or aspirate, common sense would tell you to stop eating it, whether it's within the IDDSI guidelines or not.

Using Our Time Well

When the global COVID-19 pandemic hit America, the SimplyThick sales team was forced to work from home. To keep ourselves busy — and because we had recently released a new and improved product formulation — we decided to tackle the challenge of updating our pureed food recipes. In updating the recipes, we also set out to ensure that all recipes produce foods that meet the IDDSI guidelines.

The SimplyThick team members who participated in this project came with diverse backgrounds and views. The team included five RDNs, an SLP, a certified dietary manager, two chefs, and seven salespeople. Some of them possessed extensive commercial cooking experience, while others claimed they ate most of their meals at restaurants or bought ready-to-eat options. Hopefully, the range of experience within our team bears a strong resemblance to that of home users reading this book. We hope you find the information and recipes detailed enough without finding them intimidating.

Getting Started

We received recipes from many sources — home users, commercial kitchen operators, chefs, and certified dietary managers. Our first step was to test and evaluate them all. We then sorted the recipes by food groups and assigned them to random SimplyThick sales representatives with varying kitchen skills across the country. To produce consistent results and provide easy comparisons, we decided to have everyone use the same model food processor. We chose the Cuisinart® 14-Cup Food Processor Model #DFP-14BCNY as our working model.

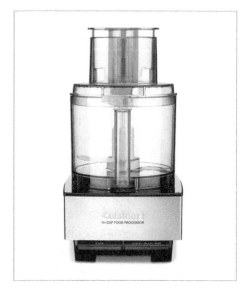

CUISINART® 14-CUP FOOD PROCESSOR

The recipe testing commenced once everyone's equipment was standardized. However, due to COVID-19, other challenges to our testing methods arose. Inventory disruptions limited the availability of test items. For instance, some fruits and vegetables were out of season so we turned to canned or frozen options. We continued to review the list of recipes over the course of several months, and test results were discussed over multiple team meetings. One repeating, problematic area the team grappled with was subjective concepts like how sticky was "too sticky?" Or, ⬇ Soft & Bite Sized uses the concept of an adult thumbnail for measurement. So the question arises: "Is your thumbnail the same size as my thumbnail?" Examples of other terms from the IDDSI descriptors that created discussion were how big or tough is a 'lump' vs. a 'bit.'

After making it through the list of foods, we started putting the details together to form easy-to-use recipes. Each recipe is written to prepare four servings. We chose four portions for each recipe for two reasons. First, four servings of most menu items fit nicely into the 14-Cup Cuisinart®. Second, part of the testing protocols we developed involved setting two servings aside and testing them after they were refrigerated or frozen and then reheated. The challenge with freezing and reheating texture-modified foods is controlling the thin liquids that may weep out after reheating the servings. Using SimplyThick® EasyMix™ fixes this problem. If four servings doesn't work for you, we've given you the proper tools to adapt the recipes as needed to fit your life situation.

We hope you find the information and recipes detailed enough without finding them intimidating.

This cookbook does not include recipes for Transitional Foods or ▼ Easy To Chew foods. We did not feel that we had the proper experience to contribute to preparing foods for these levels.

A final reminder of caution: when you prepare meals at home, your guiding principle should always be whether a particular food poses a choking risk for you or your loved one. If a food or drink causes choking — regardless of whether it is inside or outside your IDDSI designation — common sense dictates that you remove it from your menu.

We sincerely hope the information in this book provides you with new options and variety in your daily menu, as well as the knowledge and inspiration to try new techniques and recipes. We invite you to submit your feedback to cookbook@simplythick.com.

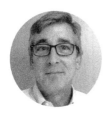

Paul Haefner

CHAPTER 3

Welcome to SimplyThick

Hello, my name is John Holahan, and I am the founder of SimplyThick, LLC. I'm also the inventor of our original product, SimplyThick.® Thank you for purchasing our cookbook.

SimplyThick is a very unique company that I've had the privilege of serving for the last 20 years. Many people might say that I "built" SimplyThick, but I really feel that all I have done is keep our focus on serving our customers. The company has grown as a result of this focus, and indeed, it has grown into the kind of place that I always believed could exist. We aren't flashy, and we don't brag very often. But we are here for you.

When asked to write a brief narrative of who we are as a company for this book, it boiled down to these all-important five points:

1. Simply put, we improve the quality of life of people with dysphagia.

2. Everything we do is in the service of improving the quality of life of people with dysphagia.

3. We provide only the best products.

4. Our primary offering is the best and most useful thickener in the world. It is a dietary aid that allows many people with dysphagia to safely manage their fluid and food consumption. As we find other relevant uses for our products, we will support them as well.

5. Because customers depend on our products for their quality of life, we don't run out of inventory.

My daily objective is to ensure that everyone in the company knows these are the core values we must live by. I don't ever want our values to be something that we simply pay lip service to or write in a book which then gathers dust. I truly see this as one of my most important jobs.

It is counter-intuitive when you don't really want your customers to need your product. It is not a particularly good day in anyone's life when their swallowing challenges have gotten to the point that they need a thickener to manage their liquids. We understand that. We have built a compassionate company — a place where you get a real, live human being on the phone when you call. A well-trained person who knows the product and can answer your questions without a script. We can't change the medical facts about your swallowing issues, but we do try to make the experience of getting your thickener and your questions answered as easy as possible.

If you ever have trouble contacting our company, try contacting me directly. My email address is john.holahan@simplythick.com, and my mobile number is (314) 422-6224. However, let me warn you that as good as I am at providing service, my customer service team is much better! Customer Service can be reached at (800) 205-7115, Monday through Friday from 8:00 AM to 6:00 PM Central.

If you would indulge me, I will take a few minutes to tell you a little bit about where SimplyThick came from and what drives all of us to be so passionate about helping you or your loved one manage a swallowing problem. The story will help you understand why there is no other product like SimplyThick® EasyMix™. Our focus on serving customers means that we insist on having the easiest to use, fastest to thicken, and most flexible product. You deserve that!

> *Everything we do is in the service of improving the quality of life of people with dysphagia.*

SimplyThick, "the company," officially came into being in May 2001. SimplyThick, "the product," was launched into the world in October 2001. But the story of SimplyThick started a few years earlier.

I was working for a small division of a large company. And it happened to be the world's largest manufacturer of xanthan gum, a commercial food thickener. One day, a co-worker called and suggested that we should sell xanthan gum to people with dysphagia because xanthan gum "gave her more time with her mother."

She went on to explain that while her mother was in hospice care, she decided that drinking beverages thickened with the thickeners available at that time was not something she wanted to do. Her mother understood the implications of not drinking liquids, yet she refused to drink them. Distraught by this, my co-worker talked about it at work, and one thing led to another. Eventually, my co-worker brought home some xanthan gum. With a blender, she began to make beverages for her mother. And her mother would drink the beverages made with xanthan gum!

The story inspired me, and I began to research the possibilities for this new market. But I soon discovered that this idea was not something that fit the business model of the international food ingredient manufacturer we were working for. As a raw material manufacturer, selling products in small retail containers was not a great fit with our business. There were already a couple of huge competitors in the dysphagia thickener market as well. Besides the corporate issues, I knew that the powder properties of xanthan gum would make it challenging for the average user to use with the tools readily available to them. We would need to find a better way to deliver the xanthan gum before it could be considered viable at scale.

We tabled the idea and set it aside.

A couple of years later, a series of events in my life brought the idea back to the forefront.

First, I began to work on an MBA while working full time. Halfway through the program, my department shut down and I lost my job.

As fate would have it, the next section of the MBA program included an Entrepreneurship class. When we looked for a business idea to incubate in class, I pitched the idea of making a better thickener for people with dysphagia. I told my classmates that we would make a xanthan gum thickener in liquid form. This would help solve all problems related to cornstarch-based powders. After a lot of quizzical looks, detailed explanations, and a lack of any other viable options, my classmates chose my idea for our class project.

We would need to find a better way to deliver the xanthan gum before it could be considered viable at scale.

As we worked on the idea, we were surprised to learn that our professor wanted real world feedback. He expected us to go out into the "real" world and get "real" answers. He said, "Why don't you call the local large teaching hospital and explain you are an MBA student with an idea you'd like their input on?" I couldn't argue with that. I was shocked when the rehab director on the other end of the phone heard my pitch and invited me to a staff meeting the next week.

At this point, the idea was strictly conceptual, as there was no prototype. But I needed one fast. I spent much of the time between that phone call and our meeting scrambling for parts, pieces, and equipment that would allow me to cobble together a functional first formulation.

We showed up with that prototype at their staff meeting and made the pitch. When I finished, there was that terrible silence hanging in the air when you don't know where the pitch landed. I'm sure it was only a second or two, but it felt like forever!

Suddenly the room came alive with questions and enthusiasm. At that moment, I knew we had struck a chord. We were really on to something! The people in that first meeting helped us immensely as we finalized our formulation and initial design.

Next, we contacted a local nursing home and repeated the process. Once again, the speech therapists were excited — even more so than the hospital group. They helped us with our product design and some data collection. They even helped us staff one of our first tradeshows!

Then, some other exciting things started to happen. I had classmates ask me if I was really going to pursue this business idea. I had a classmate tell me that if I started a company, he wanted to start it with me. I had another classmate tell me that if I started a company, he wanted to invest. Another professor heard the buzz and said that if I started a company, he wanted to invest.

However, at the time, my wife was pregnant with our first child, and I was unemployed. At this point, I also received a job offer from a large St. Louis company that would be a great reward for the MBA and included all the big company perks — healthcare, bonus, nice salary, vacation, etc.

May 2001 rolled around and we started the company to pursue the thickener idea — even though at the moment I was not yet committed to work for the start-up company. When our first child was born, my wife quit her job in order to be the primary caregiver. So yes, at this point we were both unemployed with a newborn at home.

But I had two great options in front of me — working for the start-up thickener company to help those with dysphagia or taking the safe job with great perks at the big company. But these two choices were on complete opposite ends of the job spectrum. There really was no way to make a pro and con list and see what the "right" choice would be.

I share this story with you to help convey how this company has been different since its founding. We strive to provide only the best products and the best service.

For us — my wife and me — it came down to a final discussion as we went and picked up our newborn's first photographs. Basically, we agreed that if I didn't pursue the thickener product (it didn't have a name yet), I would always wonder whether it would have been a success and if it would really have made a difference in people's lives.

In the end, my wife and I committed ourselves to the start-up thickener company, and I turned down the great offer from a huge company.

I share this story with you to help convey how this company has been different since its founding. We strive to provide only the best products and the best service. With our exceptionally high standards in mind, I challenged my team of professionals to take our product to the next level by eliminating some of the guesswork from preparing dysphagia diet foods. They have succeeded beyond my expectations and I hope you will agree that this is some of the best service we can provide for you.

Cooking for a patient with a swallowing problem is unlike anything else we do in the kitchen. Precision of texture and preparation is demanded to ensure that person's safety while eating. It is a privilege that you have the opportunity to prepare the food for your loved one; but there is also some serious responsibility. My team has done an outstanding job refining and testing each recipe. Our goal has been to ensure that every single recipe is easy and simple. Yet each one meets all the requirements of the latest IDDSI Standards.

I am proud to share this cookbook with you and your loved one. If you have any insights or feedback for us, we would love to hear from you. Feel free to send your thoughts, questions, and comments to cookbook@simplythick.com

Thanks again for trusting us to join and assist you on your dysphagia journey.

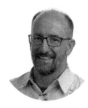

John Holahan, President, SimplyThick, LLC

CHAPTER 4

What is IDDSI and Why Are We Using It?

IDDSI is the acronym for the International Dysphagia Diet Standardisation Initiative. Rather than saying the five letters individually (I-D-D-S-I), the organization pronounces IDDSI as "ID-SEE."

The truth is that without IDDSI, this cookbook would not exist. IDDSI's gift to the world is a set of descriptors, definitions, and testing methods that allows anyone in any part of the world to be confident that prepared foods and beverages meet standardized definitions. These standardized descriptors and testing methods allowed us to develop the process we used for these recipes. And they ensure that the results meet all the requirements of the diet level.

The ability to do the testing in your own kitchen will give you the confidence that you have correctly prepared each food every time. One of the difficulties with dysphagia diets and texture-modified food preparations is the natural variability found in food from one brand to another or one day to another. Some of our recipes include notes about different experiences in our different test kitchens. This is to be expected. But the use of IDDSI test methods eliminates the guesswork and ambiguity of relying solely on descriptors. You now have quick, simple, and easy test methods that can be used to confirm you have made the food appropriate to your or your loved one's needs.

Previously published dysphagia diets often relied on lists of foods that were "allowed" or "not allowed." At first glance, this seemed to be a simple way to make the diet understandable and easy to use. However, during its development process, IDDSI recognized that many foods have properties that may change day to day, or from supplier to supplier, or after preparation and before consumption. They may not process as easily, they may get thicker or thinner, or they become sticky as they sit on a plate. An example is mashed potatoes. They may have been creamy and soft when you made them, but after sitting on a plate for an hour, they may be hard and/or sticky. Or, consider a banana. It may be too firm today, but tomorrow it will meet the IDDSI definition of "soft." Because of these very commonly occurring variable characteristics of foods, IDDSI chose a descriptive framework. Each diet level is a description of how food and liquids that meet the standard should look and behave. Under the IDDSI Framework, we never assume that a food meets the requirements of that level. Instead, we test the food after preparation to confirm that at this moment today, the way I prepared it, with the ingredients I used today, the food does meet the physical and behavioral requirements of that IDDSI level. And, the IDDSI Testing Methods are so simple and quick that we can easily monitor any changes in a food's behavior as it sits or as it is consumed.

As of this writing, IDDSI is being adopted in the health care systems of many countries. In the United States, IDDSI standards are endorsed by the American Speech-Language-Hearing Association and the Academy of Nutrition and Dietetics. The IDDSI standards are currently implemented in hospitals and long-term care communities across the country, and they have become the industry standard and established best practice.

IDDSI OVERVIEW

The most complete and up-to-date information on IDDSI is always available at www.iddsi.org. Much of the IDDSI website is generally geared to healthcare professionals, and it addresses many issues that would come up in a healthcare setting. The overview presented here is a somewhat simplified description of the IDDSI Framework specifically meant to educate consumers. If you are interested in more information, details, and research about the Framework than what is provided here, refer to their web site.

The IDDSI Framework focuses on texture irrespective of other factors such as nutritional content or taste. It is a standardisation of terminology, description, and testing methods designed to ensure foods and drinks are prepared and behave in a consistent manner. It is a set of descriptive diet levels. IDDSI defines each food texture or beverage thickness and allows for great flexibility of food and drink choices within those descriptions.

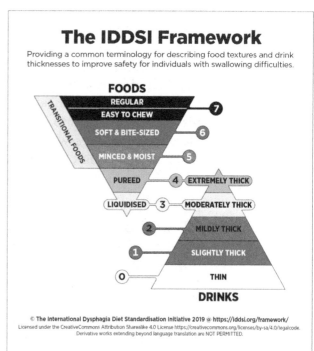

The IDDSI Framework as it currently exists is shown to the right. It includes numeric levels ranging from Level 0 for thin (regular) drinks to Level 7 for regular texture foods. And within Level 7 is a subcategory, Easy to Chew. Each level is identified with a color, a number, and a name. Any one identifier (color, number, or name) or combination thereof is enough to identify the correct diet level. The choice to offer three equal identifiers is meant to offer flexibility to clearly communicate the appropriate diet levels in a manner that best fits the operations of any health care setting. In home use, we have found that using the name of the diet level is the simplest choice.

The IDDSI Framework describes a continuum of diet levels from thin drinks to solid foods. Each level is descriptive of the characteristics and behavior of a food or drink that meets the diet level.

For the sake of consistency and clarity, we had long discussions about how to consistently communicate modified diet levels in this book. In the end, we chose to use an IDDSI numeric triangle and the diet level name. For example, ⑤ Minced & Moist.

The IDDSI Framework describes a continuum of diet levels from thin drinks to solid foods. Each level is descriptive of the characteristics and behavior of a food or drink that meets the diet level. IDDSI diet level names were also chosen to invoke a mental image of what food fitting the level should look like.

Under the IDDSI system, each person has an assigned level for their foods and another level for their drinks. ⓪ Thin drinks are unrestricted normal thin liquids while ▼ Regular food is any food without restriction. This means that the IDDSI diet levels can be used for everyone.

The IDDSI Framework consists of two pyramids. One pyramid characterizes the liquids, and the other describes solid foods. Within IDDSI and within this book, we use the words liquids, beverages, and drinks interchangeably; for a food preparation perspective, there is no difference. The base of the drink pyramid is unrestricted, everyday liquids. As you move up the pyramid, the acceptable beverages become thicker. When you reach ④ Extremely Thick, the beverages are more like a pudding than a liquid.

The general thinking when modifying drinks for swallowing problems is that thickening a liquid makes it easier to control in the mouth. Generally, as a person's motor control decreases, the beverage thickness increases. The use of the IDDSI Flow Test determines the thickness and Framework level for any beverage.

The food pyramid is upside down compared to the liquid pyramid, so its base is at the top. But just like with the drinks pyramid, the base level is unrestricted, everyday foods. Within this category is a subcategory defined as ▼ Easy to Chew. As you move down the food pyramid, the foods become more processed and refined — even to the point of being ready to swallow without any further chewing by the person with dysphagia.

The goal of modifying foods is to prepare the food to a point that mimics the person's ability to finish chewing the food and swallow it on their own. This means we substitute a food processor or other kitchen tools to complete the part of the normal chewing process that the person with dysphagia is unable to manage on their own. The goal is to let the person participate and enjoy eating as much as possible within their current physical limitation(s).

A helpful way to understand that each IDDSI level is part of our normal eating process is to imagine yourself eating a piece of cheese or soft meat. As you begin chewing, the food quickly breaks down into pieces that would be ▼6 Soft and Bite-Sized. As you continue to chew and process the food in your mouth, the food pieces become smaller and smaller and mix with your saliva until they are broken down to a ▼5 Minced and Moist level. At this point, the food is in really small pieces, is well mixed with saliva, and is almost ready to swallow. Many people without dysphagia will swallow the food at this point. And most will swallow it before processing it all the way to the next IDDSI level. However, if you continue to hold the food in your mouth and chew and process the food until it becomes smooth with no lumps, it becomes ◄4 Pureed. At this point, the food could be swallowed by almost anyone without any further chewing. However, if you continue to hold the food in your mouth long enough, it would become more and more liquid-like as more saliva is added to it. Eventually, you would have a ⅊3 Liquidised food in your mouth.

With your loved one's dysphagia diagnosis, their ability to completely chew and process food on their own has been disrupted. Using IDDSI food levels in the kitchen allows us to pre-process food they love to the point that they can take over and finish the job themselves. Stop and think about the physical ability of the person for whom you are preparing foods. Perhaps chewing is very difficult and very tiring. They can't chew for a long time. So they need their foods to be a ▼5 Minced and Moist diet. They still get to chew a little. They still get to enjoy the flavors. And they can participate in the meal. When we work together to help people enjoy their meal as independently as possible, we respect their dignity and enhance their quality of life.

An important element to keep in mind as you learn about IDDSI diet levels is that IDDSI definitions and descriptors apply to food and drink at the moment they are placed in the mouth — not necessarily when they were prepared, nor when they were put on the table at the start of the meal. Some foods are likely to change between the time you prepare them and the time they are eaten. Temperature and moisture changes can impact the characteristics of foods, so it is extremely important to pay attention as the person eats and watch for changes in food textures and

> *Using IDDSI food levels in the kitchen allows us to pre-process food they love to the point that they can take over and finish the job themselves.*

An important element to keep in mind as you learn about IDDSI diet levels is that IDDSI definitions and descriptors apply to food and drink at the moment they are placed in the mouth — not necessarily when they were prepared nor when they were put on the table at the start of the meal.

behaviors during the course of a meal. For this reason, IDDSI test methods are specifically designed to be quick and easy to use throughout a meal.

A great example that most Americans are familiar with is mashed potatoes. They may be smooth (not sticky) and wonderful when you prepare them, but 30 to 60 minutes later, they are cold and sticky. At this point, the sticky potatoes can be unsafe for people on a dysphagia diet. It is not a problem if you spot it and refresh the potatoes with some heat and a little more butter or milk to soften and smooth them again. But if you are not paying attention, the consequences can be dire.

Levels 3 and 4 are present on both the food and the drinks pyramids and are connected between the pyramids. This is to meant to communicate that the behavior and physical characteristics of the food and the beverage at these levels are very similar. ▽ Pureed foods behave the same as △ Extremely Thick liquids. ▽ Liquidised foods and △ Moderately Thick liquids also have similar physical characteristics and Framework testing standards.

It can be a little confusing to have a liquid level and a food level with the same number and color designations. However, IDDSI denotes foods with a triangle pointing downward and liquids with an upward pointing triangle. So, when you see ▽, you know that we are referring to Pureed foods. And when you see △, you know we are referring to Extremely Thick liquids. This is the same with ▽ Liquidised foods and △ Moderately Thick liquids.

Finally, we used the IDDSI Framework to guide us in developing this cookbook, and we used the IDDSI Testing Methods in testing all of our recipes. However, be aware that IDDSI has not endorsed our work in any manner. IDDSI, as an organization, owns and publishes the framework. IDDSI, as an organization, does not endorse this or any other cookbook or product. The IDDSI Framework and Descriptors are licensed under the CreativeCommons Attribution Sharealike 4.0 License.

IDDSI Test Methods

The real breakthrough that IDDSI brings to the table is the set of simple and easy test methods that almost anyone can perform anywhere. These tests use a specific plastic syringe and items found in most homes like a fork, a spoon, or chopsticks. And even if you don't have any of those, you can use your fingers with most tests! Although we will briefly review these test methods, we STRONGLY encourage you to review the IDDSI Testing Methods document reprinted in Appendix B (p. 199) or on the IDDSI website at www.iddsi.org.

The real breakthrough that IDDSI brings to the table is the set of simple and easy test methods that almost anyone can perform anywhere.

Our review of the testing methods is based on the script written by John Holahan for the IDDSI 201 webinar first presented in May 2020. If you want to watch this presentation rather than read about it, you can find it on the IDDSI YouTube Channel as part of the "What is IDDSI" playlist. Or type "IDDSI 201" into the search bar at www.youtube.com.

The overview presented here introduces the key concepts of the "IDDSI Framework Testing Methods" document. It also pulls information found in the "Complete IDDSI Framework Detailed Definitions" document. You can read these documents in the Appendix A (p. 184) or at www.iddsi.org.

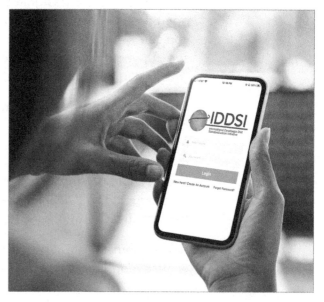

IDDSI created an app that can be downloaded to a smartphone or tablet from either the Google or Apple app store. With the app, you can download the most up-to-date information from IDDSI right onto your phone or tablet. You will be able to access key IDDSI documents and videos demonstrating these testing methods anywhere you go. It is a very effective and efficient tool.

IDDSI APP

The IDDSI test methods* are:

1. IDDSI Flow Test

2. Fork Drip Test

3. Spoon Tilt Test

4. Food Size Assessments

5. Fork Pressure Test

6. Fork/Spoon Separation Test

7. Chopstick and/or Finger Tests

IDDSI faced a dilemma regarding testing while developing the IDDSI Framework. They wondered, how can you quickly and easily test foods and drinks right at the point of consumption, anywhere in the world, at any time? There are fancy and costly pieces of equipment in laboratories that can accurately and precisely test food and drinks. But in the real world – that is, right at the point of eating or drinking – we need accessible, accurate tests to ensure that the food or drink meets all the texture and thickness criteria when consumed.

The testing methods IDDSI settled upon will answer the basic questions of how thick is "thick," how soft is "soft," and how small is "small." And all tests are based on the best available evidence. Yet they are simple, practical, and portable across ALL cultures around the world. They are also meant to be reliable and accurate.

IDDSI test methods are designed to minimize the need for personal or subjective judgement. However, you will see that some individual evaluation remains in some of these tests. Hopefully, you will recognize that every effort has been made to minimize the amount of judgement required to evaluate each food or drink.

* Since Transitional Foods are not included in this book, we have intentionally left out an IDDSI testing method that applies only to them.

1. IDDSI Flow Test

The IDDSI flow test assesses how liquids flow (or don't flow) through a syringe. This test is used to classify liquid levels 0–3: 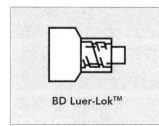 Thin, Slightly Thick, Mildly Thick, and Moderately Thick. Supplies needed to conduct this test include at least one 10 ml syringe (see below for type) and a 10-second timer.

BD Luer-Lok™

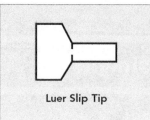
Luer Slip Tip

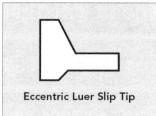
Eccentric Luer Slip Tip

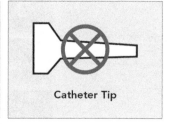
Catheter Tip

To perform this test:

1. Remove the plunger from the test syringe. Then, cover the syringe tip with your pinky finger to make a tight seal.

2. Add 10 ml of the drink you are testing to the syringe — usually using a second syringe to avoid spillage.

3. Remove your pinky finger for 10 seconds to let the drink flow out.

4. After the 10 seconds, seal the end of the syringe with your pinky again.

5. The amount of remaining liquid in the syringe will classify the IDDSI level of the liquid:

   - If less than 1 ml is remaining, the liquid is Thin.
   - If there is between 1–4 ml remaining, the liquid is Slightly Thick.
   - If there is between 4–8 ml remaining, the liquid is Mildly Thick.
   - If there is between 8–10 ml remaining, the liquid is Moderately Thick.
   - If all 10 ml remain with no drips, you have a liquid that may be Extremely Thick.

Under the IDDSI system, if you are trying to confirm a beverage is Extremely Thick, use the Fork Drip and Spoon Tilt Tests as opposed to the Flow Test, as drinks this thick will not flow through the syringe nozzle. It can be challenging to even get a liquid that is Extremely Thick loaded into the syringe. Occasionally, when making a Moderately Thick drink, you may find that it has been over-thickened and you will get a 'no-flow' or 10 ml result. In this case, you will have to dilute the beverage with some of the unthickened drink to get it back into the range of Moderately Thick drinks.

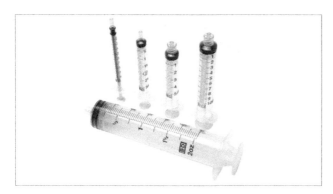

BECTON DICKINSON (BD) SYRINGES

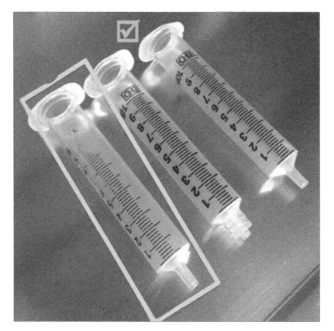

OVERUSED SYRINGES

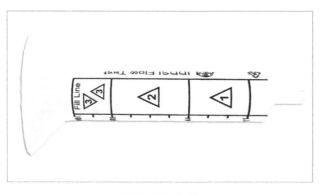

IDDSI FUNNEL

A couple of notes about the specific syringe to use for this test. There is an existing international standard on the form and shape of the syringe nozzle. But, there is some variation between manufacturers on the diameter of the syringe barrel. This will affect how much of the thickened drink flows through the syringe in 10 seconds. Therefore, it is critical to check the length of the markings from 0–10 ml on the barrel to be sure it meets the IDDSI standard length of 61.5 mm long.

If you are uncertain whether you have a compliant syringe or if you think you may have a damaged syringe, there is a quick calibration test. Fill the syringe with water to the 10 ml mark and time how long it takes for the syringe to empty. If it empties in about 7 seconds, it is appropriate to use for IDDSI Flow Testing.

The 10 ml plastic syringes come with a variety of nozzles or tips that do not affect Flow Test results. The Luer-Lok™, eccentric luer slip tip, and luer slip tip all work fine for the IDDSI Flow Test. However, the catheter tip is NOT suitable for Flow Testing because it has a different tip geometry.

You can wash and reuse syringes as long as the markings remain clear. You can see in photo to the left that the syringe on the far left is becoming difficult to read accurately. This syringe should be discarded.

IDDSI has recently released the IDDSI Funnel. It is easier to use than the 2 syringe system. You can order some at www.simplythick.com. If you prefer to find syringes, Becton Dickinson (BD) part numbers 301604, 303134, 309604, and 302995 are all known to be suitable for IDDSI Flow Testing. We have had success purchasing these via amazon.com.

2. Fork Drip Test

With the Fork Drip Test, we evaluate how liquids flow (or don't flow) through the tines of a fork. This test is used with ⚃ Moderately Thick, ⚃ Liquidised, ⚃ Extremely Thick, ⚃ Pureed, and ⚃ Minced & Moist.

For ⚃ Moderately Thick drinks and ⚃ Liquidised food, simply scoop or draw a fork through the liquid and observe how it flows through the tines. There should be a small amount that remains on top of the fork with no significant mounding, and the liquid should drip slowly or in dollops or strands through the tines. Note that you should NOT perform this test by pouring the liquid on top of the fork. This practice can lead to inconsistent results.

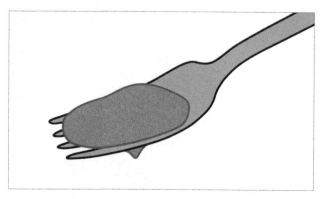

When testing an ⚃ Extremely Thick drink or a ⚃ Pureed food, the sample should sit on top of the fork tines with maybe a small tail hanging beneath (as seen in the diagram at right). But the sample does NOT flow, dollop, or drop continuously through the fork tines.

When testing for ⚃ Minced & Moist, the food should sit on top of the fork. Nothing, in particular thin liquids, should be flow or drip through the tines.

SAMPLE FOOD ON TOP OF FORK TINES

3. Spoon Tilt Test

The Spoon Tilt Test checks the cohesiveness and stickiness of a sample by evaluating how a scoop of liquid or food falls (or does not fall) off a spoon. This test is used with ▲ Extremely Thick drinks, ▼ Pureed food, and ▼ Minced & Moist food.

With this test, we are looking for a balance. We want a sample that is just tacky enough to hold its shape on the spoon, but not so sticky that it sticks to the spoon. The full spoonful must slide off the spoon as it is tilted or turned sideways. It is acceptable if a thin film remains on the spoon after the test, or if the sample spreads on the plate after it lands. The thin film remaining on the spoon after the spoon tilt test should be thin enough to see the spoon.

Note: In this test we are allowed to do a very gentle "flick" using only the fingers and the wrist to get the sample to slide off the spoon. We are NOT allowed to move the arm. This is a delicate balance that you need to be aware of. We have found success in limiting arm movement by holding our forearm with our other hand while performing this test.

Here are a couple of examples of acceptable and unacceptable tests:

In this series of photos, the sample falls off and leaves a small film.
This is acceptable.

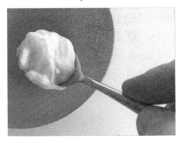 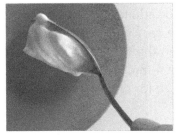 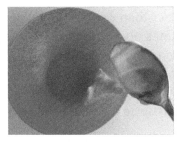

In the next series of photos, the sample looks more like peanut butter. You can see it took a lot of force to dislodge the test sample, while too much remains on the spoon. This is NOT acceptable.

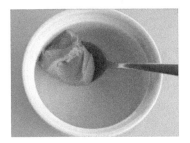 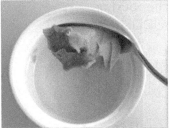 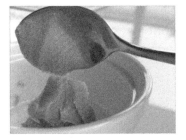

4. Food Size Assessments

To assess the size of food pieces, IDDSI relies on a fork and an adult thumbnail. These assessments are used for ▼6 Soft & Bite-Sized and ▼5 Minced & Moist.

A key aspect of preparing ▼6 Soft & Bite-Sized food is to ensure that if the piece of food is inhaled rather than swallowed, it will not be big enough to fully block you or your loved one's ability to breathe. Based on the typical size of the trachea, IDDSI requires pieces of food to be no larger than 15 mm x 15 mm x 15 mm for adults and 8 mm x 8 mm x 8 mm for children.

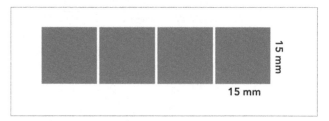

▼6 SOFT & BITE-SIZED FOOD SIZE FOR ADULTS

IDDSI has found two simple and convenient ways to measure 15 mm: the width of a typical dinner fork or a typical adult thumbnail. Before using either, please check the width of your fork or thumbnail to confirm they are the proper width. For 8 mm x 8 mm x 8 mm testing, you may have to search your kitchen for a convenient tool to use instead of a ruler.

Typically, adults without chewing and swallowing issues will chew and process food in the mouth until the individual pieces of food are between 2 mm and 4 mm before forming and swallowing a food bolus (the medical term for a soft chewed mass of food ready to swallow). ▼5 Minced & Moist requires lumps to be less than or equal to 4 mm for adults and 2 mm for children. Most standard fork tines are 4 mm apart. So, the very simple size assessment for ▼5 Minced & Moist is to ensure food fits between the tines of a fork. Please ensure that the tines of the forks in your home are 4 mm apart to properly judge this level. To test ▼5 Minced and Moist food size for children, you will have to estimate half of the distance between the tines.

In real life, food is three-dimensional. The ▼5 Minced & Moist details from IDDSI allow food to be 4 mm x 4 mm x 15 mm for adults and 2 mm x 2 mm x 8 mm for children. This allows for things like rice or chopped-up noodles to be compliant with IDDSI without more processing.

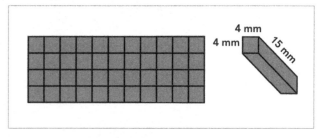

▼5 MINCED & MOIST FOOD SIZE FOR ADULTS

5. Fork Pressure Test

The Fork Pressure Test is used to evaluate the firmness of a food sample. This is used for ⑤ Minced & Moist, ⑥ Soft & Bite-Sized, and ⑦ Easy to Chew. Note that a spoon can also be used, but it is not usually recommended.

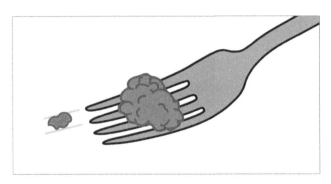

SAMPLE FOOD ON TOP OF FORK TINES

For ⑥ Soft & Bite-Sized and ⑦ Easy to Chew, press on a 15 mm x 15 mm piece of the food with your thumb just above the tines of the fork. Use just enough force so that the tip of your thumbnail blanches or turns white. The test portion should squash with ease and not return to its original shape. To be acceptable, we want to see the sample squashed, broken, or changed permanently in shape.

For ⑤ Minced & Moist, the sample should be easily mashed with just a little pressure. Also, the food should separate and come through the tines of the fork.

There are a couple of interesting notes about this test method. First, the amount of force required to blanch the thumbnail is quite consistent around the world, regardless of skin tone. Second, when the amount of pressure required to blanch the skin underneath the fingernail was measured, it was found to be almost the same as the pressure generated in the mouth when swallowing. So, as simple as it seems, the Fork Pressure Test does simulate the pressures used during swallowing.

6. Fork/Spoon Separation Test

This test uses a fork or spoon to ensure the food is easy to break down into smaller pieces while processing food in the mouth. This test is for ⑥ Soft & Bite-Sized and ⑦ Easy to Chew.

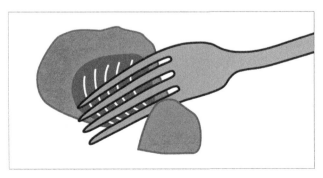

SAMPLE FOOD CUT WITH FORK

To conduct this test, use the side of a fork or a spoon to try cutting through the food with no more force than it takes to blanch the fingernail. Food separated using this gentle force passes the test.

7. Chopstick and/or Finger Tests

IDDSI is a global standard established to meet the needs of people of all ages and cultures. It includes awareness that different utensils and/or fingers are used to eat throughout the world. You will find alternative testing options using chopsticks and/or fingers in the detailed descriptors for each level, as appropriate. These alternatives are found for levels 3, 4, 5, 6, and 7EC.

Yes, even ⑶ Moderately Thick has finger-test instructions.

FINGER-TEST INSTRUCTIONS FOR ⑶ MODERATELY THICK	
Test Availability	**Standards**
Where forks are not available, Chopstick Test	Chopsticks are not suitable for this texture
Where forks are not available, Finger Test	It is not possible to hold a sample of this food texture using fingers, however, this texture slides smoothly and easily between the thumb and fingers, leaving a coating

As you can see here, chopsticks are not appropriate. However, using your fingers, this texture slides smoothly and easily between the thumb and fingers, leaving a coating. For example, some smoothies and milkshakes are moderately thick liquids that you might have experienced without additional processing.

Another example shown from the IDDSI website is from ⑸ Minced and Moist.

FINGER-TEST INSTRUCTIONS FOR ⑸ MODERATELY THICK	
Test Availability	**Standards**
Where forks are not available, Chopstick Test	Chopsticks can be used to scoop or hold this texture if the sample is moist and cohesive and the person has very good hand control to use chopsticks
Where forks are not available, Finger Test	It is possible to easily hold a sample of this texture using fingers; small, soft, smooth, rounded particles can be easily separated using fingers; the material will feel moist and leave fingers wet

You can use chopsticks to scoop or hold this texture if the sample is moist and cohesive.

Note: The person still does need to have good dexterity to properly use chopsticks. When using your fingers for this test, it is possible to easily hold the sample. And while the small, soft, smooth, rounded particles can be easily separated using fingers, the material will feel moist and leave your fingers wet.

These seven tests are all that we need to test foods and liquids as we prepare them for someone requiring a texture-modified diet.

1. IDDSI Flow Test

2. Fork Drip Test

3. Spoon Tilt Test

4. Food Size Assessments

5. Fork Pressure Test

6. Fork/Spoon Separation Test

7. Chopstick and/or Finger Tests

Not only are they quick, simple, and easy, but using them properly will ensure that you are serving food exactly as your healthcare provider has ordered. You only need to use the test methods that match the IDDSI food and drink levels recommended by your SLP.

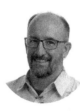

John Holahan, President SimplyThick, LLC

CHAPTER 5

Nutrition

Nutrition is important for general health. When you are sick, getting adequate nutrition is even more important. It is crucial to take in adequate calories and protein, stay hydrated, and ensure that you are getting the necessary vitamins and minerals to meet your nutritional needs.

When dysphagia is added into the mix, there is an additional need to ensure that foods and liquids can be swallowed safely. People with dysphagia may limit their food variety and volume because those foods may be difficult to swallow. This can make it difficult to reach daily nutrition goals. When this occurs, it becomes critical to develop strategies to provide adequate nutrition in spite of the reduced intake.

We want to help you enjoy and savor the foods you eat. We developed the recipes and techniques in this book to provide flavorful foods with good nutrition that will help you safely meet your nutritional needs. In addition, once you have learned the techniques, you may be able to adapt some of your own favorite recipes to meet your diet requirements.

Since there are so many excellent resources available that cover general nutrition and nutritional needs in detail, we won't cover that information here. MyPlate.gov is the consumer-friendly interpretation of the USDA's Dietary Guidelines for Americans. If you need to learn about general nutrition, this is a great place to start. However, you should be aware that the MyPlate guidelines are geared toward healthy people. They are not meant as clinical guidelines for chronic disease. Speak with your RDN about your or your loved one's specific needs.

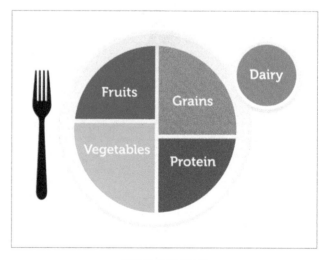

MYPLATE.GOV

The reality is that with the combination of underlying disease and dysphagia, it may become very difficult to meet all the hydration and nutrition needs without some interventions. This is when consultation with your RDN will be extremely important and especially valuable. Their training, expertise, and experience can help you and your loved one deal with the bumps in this journey. Whether your issue is lack of hydration, caloric deficits, or any number of other nutrition issues, they will be able to offer guidance on best practices and how to supplement your nutritional needs.

The following few sections include tips to help you deal with some of the most common issues encountered when someone has dysphagia.

GENERAL TIPS FOR INCREASING OVERALL CALORIES AND/OR PROTEIN*

Keep the following tips in mind to encourage greater overall consumption:

- Several small meals a day are easier to eat and digest than three large ones.

- Space meals about 2 to 3 hours apart to maximize comfort.

- Add calories to at least one food item at each meal and snack (see specific tips in the following sections).

- Eat when you feel hungry. Many people have the greatest appetite in the morning because they have not eaten all night. If this is the best meal for you, then increase calories and other nutrients in the morning and at lunch. Then, you can have a smaller dinner without losing total calories for the day.

- If you don't feel hunger or sometimes forget to eat, set a schedule of times to eat, or set a timer for reminders to eat.

- Have your favorite snacks available at all times and keep them visible as a reminder to eat.

- Eat leftovers or nutritious snacks in the afternoon and early evening to round out your day.

- Drink supplements or shakes with a snack between meals.

- Make the meal experience pleasant. Examples include dining with others, increasing the aesthetic appeal by setting the table, or using a centerpiece such as flowers.

- Breakfast-type foods are okay at any meal. Eggs are usually easy to eat and are great any time of the day.

- Save room for calorie-rich foods. Drink most fluids between meals or 30 minutes after a meal, as fluids can quickly give you a sense of fullness.

* Nutrition Care Manual®. Academy of Nutrition & Dietetics. Chicago, 2022.

Another technique to increase overall food consumption is to improve the visual appeal of the meal with an impressive presentation. It is disappointing that we often see purees and other processed foods served in an unappealing manner. We often see big, green and brown blobs of pureed foods being served. Research shows that improving the visual appearance of pureed foods by simply shaping the puree with a food form increases the amount of food consumed by a significant amount. Rush University in Chicago conducted a study about shaped purees. The study found that the patients who received shaped purees consumed an average of 500 calories more per day than those not receiving shaped purees.[1]

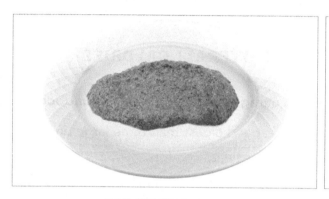

BAD PRESENTATION

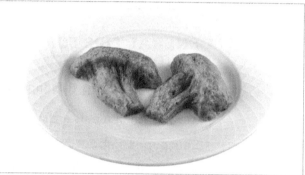

GOOD PRESENTATION

In addition, a poster session from the University of Washington found that patients who were served shaped purees vs. non-shaped purees consumed 29% more calories and 20% more protein.[2]

Although the research has only been done with pureed foods, our work with ⑤ Minced & Moist recipes has shown the benefits of food forms as well. Surprisingly, these forms do not need to look like or mimic the real food. Research has shown that simply using a geometric shape is all that is needed.[1]

It takes only a little extra time to learn to use a food form. Commercial food forms suitable for shaping ⑤ Minced & Moist and ④ Pureed foods are available online at www.dysphagia-diet.com, www.amazon.com, and www.simplythick.com/Food-Forms.

Another easy way to improve the visual appeal of the food is to use a pastry bag and different decorating tips to pipe pureed food and condiments onto a dish. It is amazing how much you can do to increase the visual appeal of a dish with this simple technique.

[1] Betz, Melanie, et al. Improved Calorie and Protein Intake Following Implementation of Formed Pureed Food. Rush University Medical Center.

[2] McBride, S., et al. "Effects of Preformed vs Unformed Puree Texture on Food Intake in Acute Care." *Journal of the Academy of Nutrition and Dietetics*, vol. 118, no. 9, 2018.

TIPS FOR INCREASING CALORIES IN RECIPES

You may find it necessary to include more calories in the food you prepare and serve to a person with dysphagia. They may not have the energy or stamina to eat as much or as long as they normally would, so increasing the number of calories in each bite may be necessary. Not all of these techniques will work with all the food in your particular diet, so choose which ones to use based on what you are preparing.

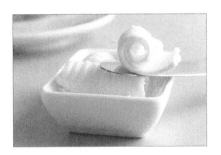

INCREASE BUTTER

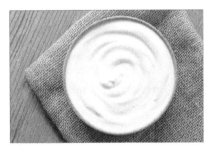

USE FULL-FAT SMOOTH YOGURT

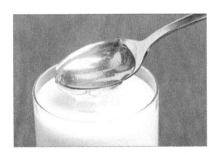

ADD HONEY TO MILK

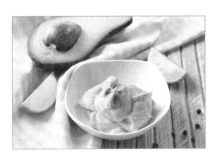

ADD MASHED AVOCADO

Increase Butter, Margarine, and Oils

- Add any of these to potatoes, rice, and cooked vegetables.
- Add any of these to soups, sauces, gravies, and casseroles.
- Use healthy oils to marinate and cook meats, chicken, and fish.

Increase Milk Products

- Use whole milk and other full-fat milk products to increase calories.
- Add sour cream to soups, potatoes, and vegetables.
- Add whipped cream to beverages and desserts.
- Use whole or 2% milk in place of water when cooking cereal and cream soups.
- Add cream cheese to vegetables.
- Use full-fat smooth yogurt (no chunks), custard or pudding, and mousse with no chunks.
- Use Half-and-Half (half whole milk, half heavy cream) instead of milk in hot cereal, milkshakes, cream soups, and sauces.
- Mix Half-and-Half with mashed potatoes to use as a substitute for milk in recipes.

Increase Sweets

- Add jelly, jam, or honey to cereals, milk drinks, yogurt, pudding, ice cream, and desserts.
- Add hot fudge to puddings.

Increase Salad Dressings and Mayonnaise

- Combine a favorite salad dressing with mayonnaise and add it to fish, meat, eggs, rice, fruits, and vegetables.

Add Avocado

- Stir mashed avocado into chocolate pudding, fruit smoothies, and cream soups.

Add Dry Pudding Mix

- Add dry pudding mix to shakes and smoothies for flavor and extra calories.

TIPS FOR INCREASING PROTEIN IN RECIPES

If you need to specifically increase the protein into a recipe, try one of these tips as appropriate for your diet.

Incorporate More Milk Products

- Use whole or 2% milk in place of water when cooking cereal and cream soups.
- Use evaporated milk, evaporated skim milk, or sweetened condensed milk instead of milk or water in recipes.
- Use Greek yogurt (no chunks) in place of regular yogurt, and add it to shakes and smoothies or serve it as a snack.
- Add cream sauces to vegetables.
- Add cheese in cooking vegetables, potatoes, rice, soups, and sauces.
- Add cottage cheese or ricotta cheese to vegetables, casseroles, eggs, and pureed dishes. Use them as a substitute for sour cream.
- Add powdered milk to cream soups, mashed potatoes, hot cereal, sauces, yogurt or milk drinks, puddings and custards, and other milk-based desserts.
- Make "double strength" milk (add ⅓ cup of nonfat powdered milk to 1 cup regular milk).

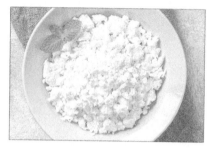

COTTAGE CHEESE

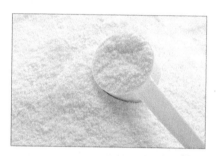

POWDERED MILK

Add Eggs

- Add eggs or liquid egg substitute to mashed potatoes, pureed vegetables, and sauces.

Increase Meat, Fish, and Poultry

- Increase the portion size of the protein part of your meal compared with side dishes.
- Blend leftover meats into soups and casseroles.

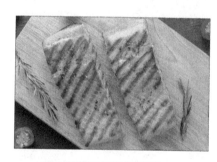

INCREASE MEAT

Add Tofu

- Blend tofu into soups, smoothies, or main course dishes.

Use Supplements and Protein Powder (after consulting with an RDN)

- Use protein powder in milk drinks and desserts, such as pudding.
- Mix protein powder with ice cream, milk, fruit, and other ingredients for a high-protein milkshake.
- Use protein shakes in place of water or milk in cooked cereals.

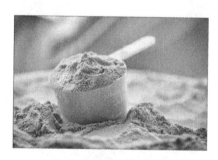

USE SUPPLEMENTS

USE OF COMMERCIAL NUTRITIONAL SUPPLEMENTS

An RDN may include a nutritional supplement into your diet if food sources or consumption are not meeting your nutritional requirements. There are many nutritional supplements on the market. Most of these nutritional supplements have 220–360 calories and 9–20g of protein per 8 oz. serving.

GENERAL GUIDELINES TO REDUCE THE CHOKING RISK FOR ADULTS WITH A DYSPHAGIA DIET

- Watch for water-thin liquids that separate from foods you prepare. These are not allowed under IDDSI diet standards.
- Eliminate large chunks or lumps.
- Avoid hard, sticky, or crunchy foods.
- Reheat foods carefully so that tough outer crusts do not form.
- Regular bread and crusts are known choking hazards and are NOT allowed under IDDSI standards.
- Avoid foods and liquids that are not recommended by your SLP, RDN, or healthcare professional.

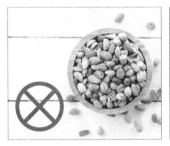 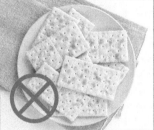 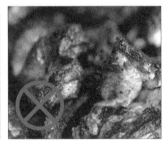 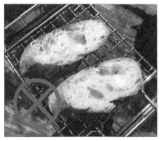

NO HARD FOODS **NO CRUNCHY FOODS** **NO OVERCOOKED FOODS** **NO REGULAR BREAD/ CRUSTS**

FOODS TO AVOID

Individuals on 6 Soft & Bite-Sized, 5 Minced and Moist, and 4 Pureed IDDSI Levels are at risk of choking. The following table, adapted from the IDDSI materials, lists the types of foods TO AVOID with some specific examples.

Food Characteristic	Examples of Foods to Avoid
Mixed thin and thick textures	Soup with pieces of food, cereal with milk
Hard or dry	Nuts, raw vegetables (e.g. carrot, cauliflower, broccoli), drycakes, bread, dry cereal
Tough or fibrous	Steak, pineapple
Chewy	Lollipops/candies/sweets, cheese chunks, marshmallows, chewing gum, sticky mashed potatoes, dried fruits, sticky foods
Crispy	Crackling, crisp bacon, cornflakes
Crunchy	Raw carrots, raw apples, popcorn

FOODS TO AVOID (continued)

Food Characteristic	Examples of Foods to Avoid
Sharp or spiky	Corn chips and crisps
Crumbly bits	Dry cake, dry biscuits
Pips, seeds	Apple seeds, pumpkin seeds, white of orange
Food with skins or outer shell	Peas, grapes, chicken skin, salmon skin, sausage skin
Food with husks	Corn, shredded wheat, bran
Bone or gristle	Chicken bones, fish bones, other bones, meat with gristle
Round, long-shaped	Sausage, grape
Sticky or gummy	Nut butter, overcooked oatmeal/porridge, edible gelatin, konjac containing jelly, sticky rice cakes
Stringy	Beans, rhubarb
Crust formed during cooking or heating	Crust or skin that forms on food during cooking or after heating, for example, cheese topping; mashed potato
Floppy	Lettuce, cucumber, baby spinach leaves
Juicy	Where juice separates from the food piece in the mouth, for example watermelon, oranges, and tomatoes.

Each IDDSI level also has specific criteria regarding the size of its pieces or lumps of food:

For 6 Soft & Bite-Sized, avoid large or hard lumps of food. Examples include casserole, fruit, vegetable, meat, pasta or any other food pieces larger than 15 mm x 15 mm.

For 5 Minced & Moist, avoid large or hard lumps of food. Examples include casserole, fruit, vegetable, meat, pasta or any other food pieces larger than 4 mm x 4 mm x 15 mm.

For 4 Pureed, avoid any lumps in pureed food or yogurt.

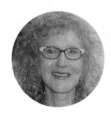

Laurie Berger, MBA, RD, LD

CHAPTER 6

The Recipes

After considerable debate and discussion, we have first organized the recipes into sections by IDDSI Levels rather than by food group.

Within those levels, you will find a stand-alone recipe for each food even though some foods process nearly identically. For example, chicken and turkey behave almost identically when processed and it was tempting to have a recipe for "chicken or turkey." However, since we are focused on teaching the user new techniques, we felt it was important to have a recipe with very specific instructions for chicken and a separate recipe with very specific instructions for turkey. This means that you may encounter similar recipes in every section of this book. And last, within each IDDSI level, the recipes are organized in the same general manner: proteins first, followed by vegetables and fruits.

Before we get to the recipes, we share additional thoughts that helped us fine-tune the recipes. We hope you enjoy this cookbook and welcome your feedback at cookbook@simplythick.com.

FOODS THAT DID NOT MAKE THE CUT

We chose not to include any recipes in this book that do not meet the IDDSI Testing Methods criteria for a full 30 minutes after preparation. Some foods meet all testing requirement immediately upon preparation, but they become too sticky upon standing. As you become more skilled in the art of texture-modified cooking, if you can serve the food immediately and your loved one can consume the food timely, then you may find that you can serve some foods that will not meet the testing criteria for a full 30 minutes.

IDDSI LEVEL DOWNWARD FLEXIBILITY

The IDDSI Framework explains the IDDSI food pyramid and its benefits. The IDDSI Framework also tells us that it is helpful to look at the levels as being "more processed" through mechanical means (and therefore being even closer to being more ready to swallow) as you move down the pyramid versus doing so by chewing. IDDSI levels start with ▼ Regular, then move to ⑥ Soft & Bite-Sized, to ⑤ Minced & Moist, and finally to ④ Pureed. What this means is that you can be safely served food from a lower level in the IDDSI pyramid than what you were prescribed. And this is when the flexibility of IDDSI levels proves to be exceptionally handy.

For example, a pork chop that is cut into bite-sized pieces for a ⑥ Soft & Bite-Sized meal is almost certainly not going to be soft enough to pass the IDDSI Fork Pressure Test. But when it is processed to ⑤ Minced & Moist with some gravy, you can serve it in place of a ⑥ Soft & Bite-Sized portion.

It is crucial to remember that this works ONLY when moving down the food pyramid. For example, if you are on a ④ Pureed diet, you can ONLY use recipes from the ④ Pureed section. But if you are on a ⑤ Minced & Moist diet, you can use recipes from the ④ Pureed section AND the ⑤ Minced & Moist section.

EQUIPMENT

When our team started testing and refining recipes, we received a wide range of results. We learned that the size and model of food processor, as well as details such as blade sharpness and speed, could make significant differences in the result of each recipe.

The Cuisinart® 14-Cup Food Processor Model No. DFP-14BCNY was used successfully when conducting several tests. The machine received great reviews and worked well for our testers.

We also used several Ninja® products with great success. The model BN601 is a little smaller bowl than the Cuisinart, but it worked well in our tests.

No matter which food processor you use, if you notice that the blade is not sharp enough or does not spin fast enough, check the food for lumps or pieces of bone, cartilage, or sinew. Remove any unwanted pieces and re-process the food if necessary.

Having a blender or food processor bowl that is the right size for the number of portions of food you are preparing is vital. If there is too much, or too little, food in the bowl, the machine will not process effectively. A good rule of thumb for best results is that the food processor bowl should not be more than half full. Once you have the batch size and the machine properly matched, you will likely see the entire contents of the processor or blender 'rolling' or 'working' together. The contents will repeatedly turn into the blade assembly to maximize efficient processing. If there is not enough food in the processor to work into the blade effectively, you will spend a lot of time scraping food off the side of the bowl. Also, cutting up large pieces of food before placing them in the food processor will produce pieces that are more consistently uniform in size more quickly.

All of the recipes in this book are properly sized to process efficiently in the Cuisinart® 14-Cup Food Processor Model No. DFP-14BCNY. If you have a different sized processor, you may need to adjust the quantities.

Other equipment we found helpful when starting to expand recipes, especially with garnishes or small but flavorful ingredients, include a mortar and pestle, a ricer (for squeezing water out of vegetables), a mesh strainer or a cheesecloth, and a sharp kitchen knife that you are comfortable and confident with. Many of our testers recommend using a pastry bag and tip (the type used for decorating cakes) to store and shape ④ Pureed and ⑤ Minced & Moist foods. Other tools that help with portion control, baking, and shaping foods include: cookie cutters, muffin cups, silicone food molds, squeeze bottles, ice cream scoops, zip-style plastic bags, and ice cube trays. We recommend reading through the recipes first before buying anything in order to determine which might be helpful to you. It should be noted that we used food forms when preparing food for photographs in this cookbook.

PROTEINS / MEATS

As already mentioned, many of the protein or meat recipes are very similar. For example, we found the process, instructions, and cautions were identical with chicken and turkey. As tempting as it was, we chose not to combine these two items into one recipe. We felt that the simplicity of a recipe for each meat would offer the clearest presentation for those new to this method of preparation. One overriding caution with the protein part of your meal is to make sure no bits of bone, gristle, or cartilage make it onto the plate. These components often lead to choking.

We use the term "stock" throughout our recipes. Stock is the shortened version of cooking stock and is another term for broth. The terms "stock" and "broth" are used interchangeably at SimplyThick. We also consider the different types of stock and broth to be interchangeable. For example, depending on the base protein called for in a recipe, you may be asked to add thickened beef stock, chicken stock, fish stock, or another type. As the actual stock used has little flavor impact on the final food, do not feel bound to using just one specific type. If you were preparing fish to ④ Pureed, for example, and did not have fish stock, you could use thickened vegetable stock or thickened water as a substitute.

We are occasionally asked about using thickened water versus assorted stocks for different dishes, especially in licensed healthcare settings that make a high volume of modified meals. In many of those facilities, patients have a lot of menu options, and the kitchen has a limited amount of time and staff. Using thickened water as a safe, 'no flavor' option for all menu items is efficient and popular. On rare occasions, we have received feedback that a surveyor "discourages adding water to recipes as it may reduce nutritional density." In general, the addition of 0–2 tablespoons of thickened liquid per portion is not sufficient enough to adversely affect patient outcomes.

In contrast with healthcare locations, there are 'at-home' users that make 4 to 6 portions of meat or fish at a time. They refrigerate or freeze those portions and reheat them when needed. Using their valuable input, we incorporated storing and reheating into our recipe development process.

We found that when reheating frozen meat that was processed without thickened stock, "water-thin liquids" were often released. Our testing found that using stock thickened with SimplyThick® EasyMix™ was very effective in preventing this from happening. We tried other thickeners available at home with much less success. We also found that the use of SimplyThick® EasyMix™ in ▽4 Pureed recipes prevented the formation of a dry crust during reheating, which would fail IDDSI testing methods.

VEGETABLES

Many vegetables weep water-thin liquids either as part of the cooking process or as a processed vegetable itself. As a first step in combatting this, we recommend draining or expressing the moisture from the vegetables. This can be achieved easily with a ricer.

For the most part, our testers found it easy to bring vegetables that had been refrigerated or frozen back to a safe and palatable temperature. The main challenge when reheating is to make sure the sample does not weep water-thin liquids, which are not allowed under the IDDSI Framework. In many cases after reheating, it may be necessary to remove any water-thin liquid or even add some ▲4 Extremely Thick stock.

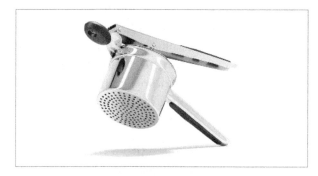

RICER

Vegetables bring a fibrous or stringy component to the mix, which will in general disqualify some items from some being served at some IDDSI levels. Snow peas and sugar snap peas are examples of this. However, sometimes we can aid the mechanical breakdown of such items by cooking them to a very well-done state. Even then, the only way to deconstruct them so they can pass IDDSI ▽4 Pureed testing is to grind them with a mortar and pestle to break down the tough or stringy components.

For example, when putting a lemon caper butter sauce together for a ▲4 Pureed baked fish, one tester used the mortar and pestle to first make a paste out of the capers. The mechanical action of the grinding broke down the outer skin and the rest of the caper. The reward was a 'caper paste' that could be rolled into small rounds placed onto the fish puree and have both items pass ▲4 Pureed tests.

As your comfort and skills increase, you may find that different tools work better for you in some scenarios than others. For example, we can achieve ▼5 Minced & Moist with many vegetables using a knife (instead of a food processor) to get all pieces to the correct size and a small amount of ▲4 Extremely Thick stock to control thin liquids. For our testers, the deciding factors on which tool to use revolved around which vegetable and how many portions were being prepared. On one occasion, a tester used a knife to cut green beans to ▼5 Minced & Moist in less than two minutes for one portion. But on a separate occasion, the same tester began with a knife on four portions of cooked carrots. After five minutes of knife work, they gave up, scraped the entire cutting board of carrots into the food processor, and was completely finished 10 seconds later.

As you progress, you can also consider mincing vegetables before the cooking process for a more evenly sized finished product. You may find some foods that turn out better when chopped, minced or pureed before preparation while others turn out better when altered after the cooking process.

FRUITS

The main challenge for most fruits is that nature puts a lot of water-thin liquid into them. We must work to lessen, or control, it. Watermelon and cantaloupe are examples of fruits with very high percentages of water. There is no amount of thickener that will keep them under control for the entire 30-minute length of the IDDSI testing. Instead of trying to find a way to consume them as whole foods, many of our longtime customers will consume these types of high-water content fruits in smoothies made to a thickness level appropriate to their needs.

Another challenge is that many fruits have seed pods, pips, or inherent fibrous tissue that are a constant threat to a safe and controlled swallow. Pineapple and mandarin oranges are good examples. The construction of a pineapple is such that there a lot of little pods or pips that make up the fruit of the pineapple. The combination of thin liquid, fibrous tissue, and sweetness (which may produce excessive saliva) makes pineapple one of the most common fruit people choke on. We could not get pineapple to pass ▲4 Pureed requirements for these exact reasons. We specifically recommend constant direct supervision for the entire meal if pineapple is on the menu for any of the texture-modified diets. To safely consume pineapple or mandarin oranges, we suggest appropriately thickening strained juice versions of the fruit.

It would be impossible to construct a consummate list of all fruits and their traits. For this reason, we recommend extreme caution when working with all fruits. Always be on the lookout for the same qualities mentioned above that put pineapple and mandarin oranges on the forbidden fruit list.

SWEETS

We tested all manner of cookies, cakes, and brownies while trying to achieve a passable version for ④ Pureed and ⑤ Minced & Moist (typically the most challenging diet textures to achieve with desserts). We were unsuccessful. By the time we deconstructed the dessert in question and put it back together, it was obvious that a chocolate milkshake or a creamy pudding would have been a better place to start and finish. We tested a variety of cookies, from Thin Mints to homemade Snickerdoodles. The results made it clear there was not a practical way to write a functional recipe for those items. Thus, our feedback on dessert is similar to 'fruits' in that making an appropriately thickened shake or smoothie can solve the craving. However, we do continue to work to find an appropriate method to transform desserts. If you find a solution you wish to share with us, please email us at cookbook@simplythick.com.

"THE NATURALS"

The IDDSI Framework allows everyone to have ④ Pureed foods without restriction. Therefore, any foods that naturally qualify as ④ Pureed are safe for everyone texture-wise.

One of the effects of this project was that for many of our testers, the work was always with us. For example, the innocent spouse of one tester was attempting to prepare guacamole for herself when our tester moved her aside to instead test a slice of ripe avocado. It was successfully smashed into ④ Pureed with a fork in 10–15 seconds and then was successfully tested to confirm that it was, indeed, a ④ Pureed food. The tester noted, "Before I got involved in testing for this cookbook, I did not pay very much attention to these foods. Now, it's about all I look for."

> "Before I got involved in testing for this cookbook, I did not pay very much attention to these foods. Now, it's about all I look for."

Many foods fit into ④ Pureed level in their natural state, or 'as is.' These foods include: yogurt (without pieces of fruit), canned pumpkin, pumpkin pie without the crust, many variations of pudding, flan, and panna cotta. Bananas and avocados can both be easily mashed to ④ Pureed consistency. On the savory and spicy side, many variations of hummus and vegetable dips can qualify for ④ Pureed foods with little to no modification.

RICE AND PASTA

Pasta and rice are essential to a wide assortment of staple dishes all over the globe. And, unfortunately, rice and pasta top of the list of everyday menu items that are difficult to prepare in a manner that will pass testing for ▽4 Pureed. They also regularly fail ▽5 Minced & Moist and ▽6 Soft & Bite-Sized because they are too sticky.

The challenge we regularly faced with rice or pasta is the inherent starchiness of wheat and rice, which results in the food becoming stickier as it sits after preparation. This is most difficult at the ▽4 Pureed level, but it is often just as relevant at ▽5 Minced & Moist and ▽6 Soft & Bite-Sized. The evaluation standard we used for gauging success or failure was in line with IDDSI guidance that food should be evaluated when prepared and again at 15 and 30 minutes later. We had many apparent successes that would fail after sitting out for 30 minutes.

We had testers try pureeing by adding water, butter, oil, acidic liquids, and more. We tried pasta made from chickpeas with no success. We tried overcooking the pasta and double rinsing with no success. The result of our testing is that trying to convert everyday rice and pasta to ▽4 Pureed was a fail.

We did have some success with macaroni and cheese at ▽5 Minced & Moist and ▽6 Soft & Bite-Sized when we modified the recipe a bit. First, we ran the dry macaroni noodles in the food processor to break them into small pieces before cooking. We rinsed the pasta after cooking. And then we thinned the cheese sauce by adding a little extra butter or oil. But we did not achieve a consistently successful ▽4 Pureed version.

Finally, during the editing stages of this cookbook, we found a solution for pasta! It involves a combination of excess cooking water, long cooking times and immediately chilling the pasta BEFORE processing. We are proud to be able to include these recipes in this edition of our cookbook.

▽5 **MINCED & MOIST MAC & CHEESE (PG. 150)**

We continue to search for a solution for rice, and we know that IDDSI has working groups looking at this question as well. You can check www.iddsi.org for the latest information.

BREAD

In the research behind the IDDSI Framework, it was found that bread is an everyday food that can pose a significant choking risk. A number of coroners' reports found bread in obstructed airways.

You can confirm the issue yourself by simply taking a small piece of bread and trying to "chew" it without using your teeth. Try to process it with your tongue only and you will likely find that it becomes sticky, may stick to the roof or your mouth, or could form a sticky ball in your mouth. The point is that without the ability to chew and process bread in your mouth, bread can form a large mass that can be very difficult to swallow properly.

It was a very difficult decision for them, but IDDSI decided to NOT include "regular" bread in its Framework.

For decades in the commercial healthcare kitchen, RDNs have worked to make a safe bread by pouring thickened milk or water on bread with little to no success. On occasions where they have come close to meeting the IDDSI criteria, they still ended up with cold wet bread that is widely unacceptable.

Our testing of bread for this cookbook led us down a different path. Unsatisfied with current practices, our team was not ready to give up on bread. They found some recipes and our testers started working with them. Some recipes were for bread pudding, which encouraged us that we could get enough of the 'stickiness' out of the bread while keeping enough of the texture and flavor to still call it bread. We conducted tests and more tests, using different ingredients, ratios of ingredients, and cooking methods. After four months of testing and tweaking, we came up with a recipe for a baked 'fortified bread' that meets the IDDSI Framework for ▽4 Pureed and is thus acceptable for ▽5 Minced & Moist and ▽6 Soft & Bite-Sized diets as well.

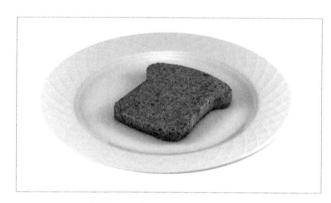

▽4 **PUREED BREAD (PG. 60)**

After testing the recipe in healthcare locations across the U.S. and receiving positive feedback, we proudly released the recipe widely in June 2021. The recipe is included in this book.

◢ EXTREMELY THICK LIQUIDS

Processing solid food with your mouth involves reducing the food to smaller pieces and mixing the food with saliva to prepare it for swallowing. This natural process is the same as mechanically processing foods to conform to IDDSI standards. The mechanical process involves cutting the food into smaller pieces and manually managing the liquids in the food.

In our recipes, we use ◢ Extremely Thick liquids for a few reasons. First, they work! Secondly, they have minimal impact on the taste with the small amount that is used.

We chose to use thickened cooking stock — be it vegetable, beef, chicken, or fish — rather than water in our recipes for the simple reason that we felt stock would dilute the flavor the least. But if you don't have any stock available, you can always use thickened water.

When you look around your kitchen, you will notice several products that are naturally ◢ Extremely Thick right off the shelf. Yogurt, ketchup, and barbeque sauce immediately come to mind. Any of these can be substitutes for ◢ Extremely Thick Stock in our recipes. However, they are not all equally interchangeable. For example, a barbeque sauce mixed into a pulled pork would be enjoyable, but yogurt mixed into the same pulled pork may not be.

Our final message to you before you head into your kitchen is to be flexible and creative! We hope that we have created an easy-to-follow roadmap for you or your loved one to follow that leads to simple, nourishing, and enjoyable meals.

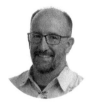

John Holahan, President SimplyThick, LLC

EXTREMELY THICK

Thickened Sauces, Dressings & Condiments

LEVEL 4 – EXTREMELY THICK

We eat with our eyes. We have all heard this over the course of our lives. Often, the meal presentation and its garnishes can make all the difference in the world. Poorly plated and garnished food may sit uneaten. But well-presented food can encourage consumption. Condiments, dipping sauces, or a side of Ranch Dressing are expected with some dishes. Or perhaps a sauce or gravy is expected on top of the dish when served. Presenting the texture-modified food in a way that you or your loved one are accustomed to helps to improve palatability and consumption.

If we review a standard offering like pureed barbeque chicken, we realize that you can prepare and serve it in many ways. You could use barbecue sauce as the lubricating liquid during the pureeing process. This will incorporate the barbecue sauce throughout the chicken. You could also put a barbecue sauce thickened to ⚠ Extremely Thick on top of pureed chicken. Or you could have some barbecue sauce thickened to ⚠ Extremely Thick served on the side of pureed chicken as a dipping sauce. All of these approaches are acceptable and appropriate. But the best option for you depends on how you or your loved one likes their barbecue chicken. The techniques and processes in this book are intended to give you confidence, regardless of how you prepare and serve a meal. Our goal is that you or your lovedone have food of the correct texture and consistency.

THE RECIPES

Basic Sauce

Buffalo Sauce

Marinara Sauce

Extremely Thick Stock

Ken's Steak House® Ranch Dressing

Ken's Steak House® Chunky Blue Cheese Dressing

ADDITIONAL TESTING RECOMMENDATIONS

There are likely many natural ⊿ Extremely Thick options in the contents of your refrigerator door and stash of condiments. These include Heinz® ketchup, McDonald's® honey mustard dipping sauce, Hellman's® mayonnaise, and light mayonnaise. There is also tartar sauce (strain out minced pickles if necessary), Grey Poupon® Dijon mustard, and Thousand Island dressing (strain out minced pickles if necessary).

Many condiments are water-thin or just slightly thicker than water. Consider soy sauce, balsamic vinegar, and assorted salad dressings. We recommend testing these items with the IDDSI test methods to confirm that they respond to thickener as expected and are safe to consume.

Lastly, for ▽ Pureed and ▽ Minced & Moist foods, we strongly recommend a meticulous examination and observation when testing chili con queso and cheese-based sauces. Besides the other criteria, the sauce should not be 'too sticky' at the 15-minute and 30-minute intervals. We could not find a commercial cheese sauce that would meet IDDSI requirements for ▽ Pureed food because they were 'too sticky' at the 15- and/or 30-minute markers.

Basic Sauce

NOTES

Follow this recipe to process basic sauces to meet IDDSI ⚠4 Extremely Thick guidelines for adults.

This recipe can be used on any type of sauce.

DIRECTIONS

1. Strain the sauce to remove solid chunks, or put in a blender and process until smooth. For small quantities, consider using a mortar and pestle for more control and less cleanup.
2. Add one 6g packet of SimplyThick® EasyMix™ or 1 pump stroke from a bottle of SimplyThick® EasyMix™ per ounce of sauce you are thickening.
3. Mix briskly for 30–60 seconds.
4. Evaluate for compliance with ⚠4 Extremely Thick guidelines:
   a. Scoop some with a fork.
      i. It should sit in a mound or a pile above a fork.
      ii. Small amounts may flow through and form a tail below the fork.
      iii. It should not dollop or flow continuously through the fork tines.
   b. Scoop some with a spoon.
      i. It should hold its shape on the spoon but is not firm and sticky.
      ii. It should fall off the spoon when turned sideways and gently flicked.
5. If it fails these tests, return to Step 2.
6. If it passes these tests, you are done.

Buffalo Sauce

INGREDIENTS

- 6 oz. of buffalo sauce
- 24g SimplyThick®
  EasyMix™—depending on the
  exact SimplyThick product(s)
  you have available to you this
  will be:
  - 4 strokes from a pump
    bottle or;
  - 6 ▲1 Slightly Thick packets
    (4g) or;
  - 4 ▲2 Mildly Thick packets
    (6g) or;
  - 2 ▨ Moderately Thick
    packets (12g)

DIRECTIONS

1. Combine sauce and SimplyThick® EasyMix™ in a bowl.
2. Mix for 30–60 seconds.
3. Test for compliance with ▲4 Extremely Thick guidelines:
   a. Scoop some with a fork.
      i. It should sit in a mound or a pile above a fork.
      ii. Small amounts may flow through and form a tail below the fork.
      iii. It should not dollop or flow continuously through the fork tines.
   b. Scoop some with a spoon.
      i. It should hold its shape on the spoon but is not firm and sticky.
      ii. It should fall off the spoon when turned sideways and gently flicked.
4. If it fails these tests, add 1 more packet or pump stroke of SimplyThick® EasyMix™ and return to step 2.
5. If it passes these tests, you are done.

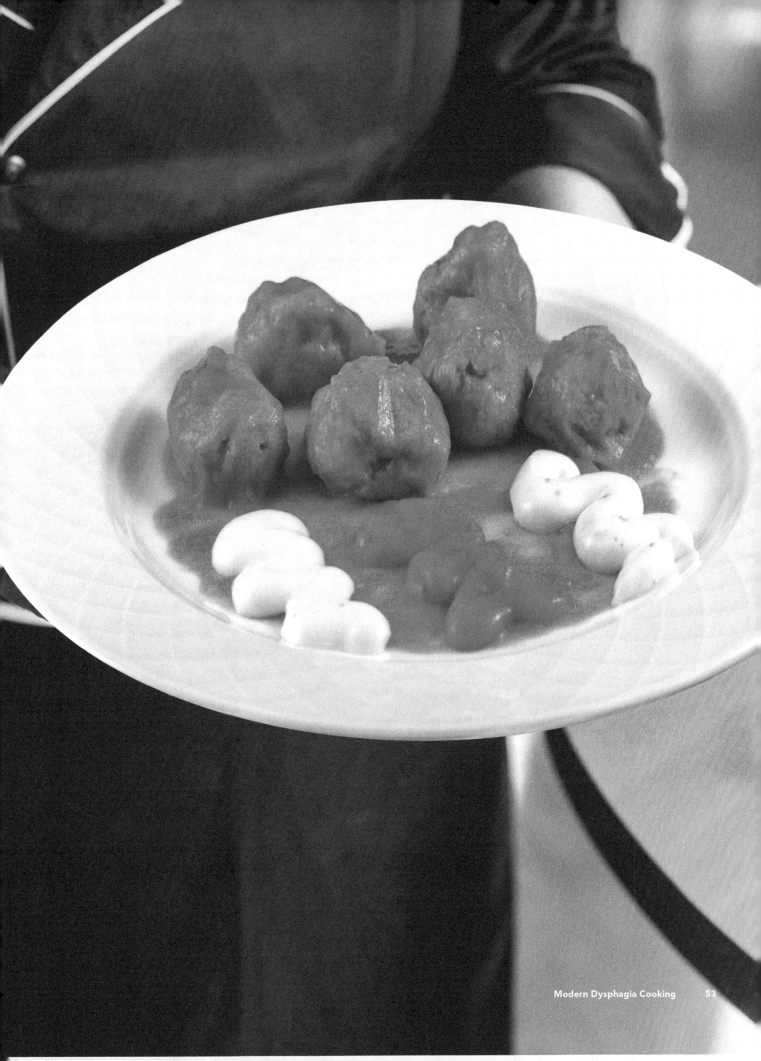

Marinara Sauce

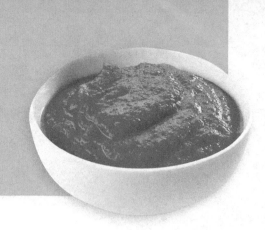

INGREDIENTS

- 24 oz. jar of marinara, spaghetti, or other red sauce or homemade equivalent
- 24g SimplyThick® EasyMix™—depending on the exact SimplyThick product(s) you have available to you this will be:
  - 4 strokes from a pump bottle or;
  - 6 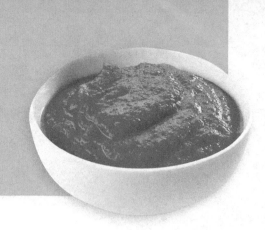 Slightly Thick packets (4g) or;
  - 4 Mildly Thick packets (6g) or;
  - 2 Moderately Thick packets (12g)

NOTES

Whether you are starting from a store-bought or a homemade marinara or other red sauce, preparing an Extremely Thick Marinara Sauce is quick and simple. Although this recipe uses a typical retail sized jar, it is easy to adapt to any quantity of sauce.

There are 2 considerations as you prepare an Extremely Thick Marinara or other red sauce:

First, any Extremely Thick liquid should be free of significant bits and pieces — it should be smooth. Onion, tomato, garlic and other ingredients can be intentionally left as large pieces and are not suitable for use as-is. They will need to be processed smooth.

Second, many sauces will need a little extra thickener to get it thick enough to meet the Extremely Thick standards. The general rule of thumb is to expect to use 1g of SimplyThick® EasyMix™ per 1 oz. of sauce. But as always, rely on your test results.

A special note on measuring thickness — sauces with bits and pieces, even when processed smooth, may not be suitable for the IDDSI Flow Test. The small bits can plug the nozzle of the syringe and give inaccurate readings. Rely on spoon and fork tests to ensure the proper thickness.

DIRECTIONS

1. Add sauce to food processor with a sharp blade.
2. Put cover on processor.
3. Run processor for 20 seconds.
4. Open processor and inspect sauce:
   a. Remove any obviously undercooked, tough or stringy pieces.
   b. Scrape sauce off the side of processor bowl.
5. Add SimplyThick® EasyMix™.
6. Put cover on processor.
7. Using approximately 20 second intervals, run processor as long as necessary to eliminate all lumps:
   a. Remove cover and scape sides after each interval of processing.
   b. Typically, 1–2 rounds of processing and scraping will be needed.
8. If you cannot process to smooth, remove obvious lumps with a spoon.
9. Evaluate to ensure compliance with IDDSI Extremely Thick requirements:
   a. No lumps and no separated water-thin liquids.
   b. Liquid sits on a mound above a dinner fork but does not drip or flow continuously through the fork.
   c. Holds shape on a spoon, and slides off a teaspoon with little left.
   d. Should not be firm or sticky.
10. Add to properly prepared pasta and serve or store in refrigerator for later use.

Extremely Thick Stock

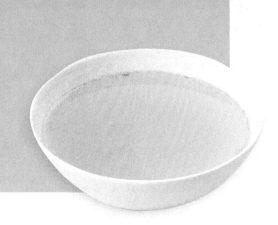

INGREDIENTS

- 8 oz. of cooking stock—vegetable, beef, chicken, fish, pork, etc.
- 48g SimplyThick® EasyMix™—depending on the exact SimplyThick product(s) you have available to you this will be:
  - 8 strokes from a pump bottle or;
  - 12 ⚠️ Slightly Thick packets (4g) or;
  - 8 ⚠️ Mildly Thick packets (6g) or;
  - 4 ⚠️ Mildly Thick bulk packets (48g) or;
  - 4 ⚠️ Moderately Thick packets (12g)

NOTES

⚠️ Extremely Thick Stock is the primary tool you use as you prepare food throughout this cookbook. It will lubricate, blend and hold the food together. If there are water-thin liquids expressed by a fruit or vegetable, the ⚠️ Extremely Thick Stock will thicken the free liquid. If a processed meat is too crumbly or dry, the ⚠️ Extremely Thick Stock will bring it together and lubricate the meat so it will not be sticky.

We have chosen to thicken cooking stock instead of water because we want to dilute the food with something more substantial than water—even though it is only by a small amount. Using cooking stock adds a little flavor and a few calories.

Generally, depending on your personal taste preferences, you can use any type of cooking stock, thicken it to ⚠️ Extremely Thick and use it with any recipe. You can choose to use vegetable stock with meat or use beef stock with chicken or vegetables. The goals of using ⚠️ Extremely Thick Stock are to facilitate the proper preparation of food to IDDSI guidelines and to achieve great taste.

DIRECTIONS

Hand Mix Directions:
1. Add 8 oz. of stock to a mixing bowl.
2. Add 48g of SimplyThick® EasyMix™.
3. Stir briskly for 30–60 seconds (until very thick).
4. Evaluate to ensure compliance with IDDSI ⚠️ Extremely Thick requirements:
   a. No lumps and no separated water-thin liquids.
   b. Liquid sits on a mound above a dinner fork but does not drip or flow continuously through the fork.
   c. Holds shape on a spoon, and slides off a teaspoon with little left.
   d. Should not be firm or sticky.
5. Pour/scrape into a squeeze bottle or other suitable container.
6. Mark the bottle with expiration date of stock or SimplyThick® EasyMix™, whichever comes first.
7. Store in refrigerator for later use.
8. Discard at expiration date.

Shaking Directions:
1. Add 8 oz. of stock to a container that can be closed tightly.
2. Add 48g of SimplyThick® EasyMix™.
3. Cover and shake for 10 seconds.
4. Evaluate to ensure compliance with IDDSI ⚠️ Extremely Thick requirements:
   a. No lumps and no separated water-thin liquids.
   b. Liquid sits on a mound above a dinner fork but does not drip or flow continuously through the fork.
   c. Holds shape on a spoon, and slides off a teaspoon with little left.
   d. Should not be firm or sticky.
5. Mark the bottle with expiration date of stock or STEM, whichever comes first.
6. Store in refrigerator for later use.
7. Discard at expiration date.

Ken's Steak House® Ranch Dressing

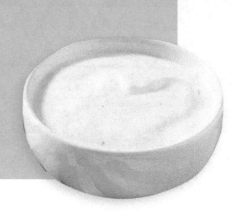

INGREDIENTS

- 4 oz. Ken's Steak House® Ranch Dressing
- 12g SimplyThick® EasyMix™— depending on the exact SimplyThick product(s) you have available to you this will be:
  – 2 strokes from a pump bottle or;
  – 3 ⚠ Slightly Thick packets (4g) or;
  – 2 ⚠ Mildly Thick packets (6g) or;
  – 1 ⚠ Moderately Thick packets (12g)

DIRECTIONS

1. Combine dressing and SimplyThick® EasyMix™ in a bowl.
2. Mix for 45 seconds.
3. Test for compliance with ⚠ Extremely Thick guidelines:
   a. Scoop some with a fork.
      i. It should sit in a mound or a pile above the fork.
      ii. Small amounts may flow through and form a tail below the fork.
      iii. It should not dollop or flow continuously through the fork tines.
   b. Scoop some with a spoon.
      i. It should hold its shape on the spoon but is not firm and sticky.
      ii. It should fall off the spoon when turned sideways and gently flicked.
4. If it fails these tests, add 1 more packet or pump stroke of SimplyThick® EasyMix™ and return to step 2.
5. If it passes these tests, you are done.

Ken's Steak House® Chunky Blue Cheese Dressing

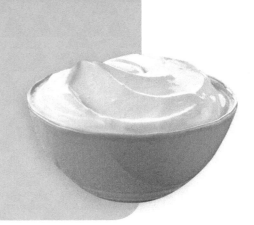

INGREDIENTS

- 4 oz. Ken's Steak House® Chunky Blue Cheese Dressing
- 24g SimplyThick® EasyMix™— depending on the exact SimplyThick product(s) you have available to you this will be:
  - 1 stroke from a pump bottle or;
  - 2 ▲ Slightly Thick packets (4g) or;
  - 1 ▲ Mildly Thick packets (6g)

DIRECTIONS

1. Use a strainer to catch and remove blue cheese chunks. Or, using a mortar and pestle, mash blue cheese chunks into dressing until smooth.
2. Combine dressing and SimplyThick® EasyMix™ in a bowl or mortar and pestle.
3. Mix for 30–60 seconds.
4. Test for compliance with ▲ Extremely Thick guidelines:
   a. Scoop some with a fork.
      i. It should sit in a mound or a pile above a fork.
      ii. Small amounts may flow through and form a tail below the fork.
      iii. It should not dollop or flow continuously through the fork tines
   b. Scoop some with a spoon.
      i. It should hold its shape on the spoon but is not firm and sticky.
      ii. It should fall off the spoon when turned sideways and gently flicked.
5. If it fails these tests, add 1 more packet or pump stroke of SimplyThick® EasyMix™ and return to step 2.
6. If it passes these tests, you are done.

PUREED

LEVEL 4 – PUREED

Description/characteristics

- Usually eaten with a spoon (a fork is possible)
- Cannot be drunk from a cup because it does not flow easily
- Cannot be sucked through a straw
- Does not require chewing
- Can be piped, layered or molded because it retains its shape, but should not require chewing if presented in this form
- Shows some very slow movement under gravity but cannot be poured
- Falls off spoon in a single spoonful when tilted and continues to hold shape on a plate
- No lumps
- Not sticky
- Liquid must not separate from solid

Physiological rationale for this level of thickness

- If tongue control is significantly reduced, this category may be easiest to control
- Requires less propulsion effort than 5 Minced & Moist, 6 Soft & Bite-Sized and 7 Regular Easy to Chew but more than 3 Liquidised and 3 Moderately Thick
- No biting or chewing is required
- Increased oral and/or pharyngeal residue is a risk if too sticky
- Any food that requires chewing, controlled manipulation or bolus formation are not suitable
- Pain on chewing or swallowing
- Missing teeth, poorly fitting dentures

Although descriptions are provided, use IDDSI Testing methods to decide if the food meets IDDSI 4 Pureed guidelines for adults.

THE RECIPES

Whole Wheat Bread

Toasted Whole Wheat Bread

Toasted English Muffins

Cinnamon Raisin Bread

Toasted Cinnamon Raisin Bread

Refrigerated Cinnamon Rolls

Pancakes from Mix

Frozen Pancakes

Frozen Waffles

Beef (Steak or Roast)

Ground Beef

Shredded Beef

Meatloaf

Meatballs

Ham

Pulled Pork

Pork Chops or Pork Loin

Chicken

Boneless Buffalo Chicken Bites

Turkey

Breaded Fish or Fish Sticks

Sauteed Fish

Scrambled Eggs

Egg Salad

Potato Salad

Chicken Salad

Tuna Salad

Coleslaw

Mashed Potatoes

Carrots

Cauliflower

Broccoli

Butternut Squash

Green Beans

Peas

Spinach

Peaches

Pears

Buttered Noodles

Homemade Shells & Cheese

Velveeta® Shells & Cheese Original

Spaghetti & Meatballs

Chocolate Raspberry Parfait

Lemon Parfait

Whole Wheat Bread

NOTES

This is the basic ④ Pureed bread recipe. All of our other ④ Pureed bread recipes are modifications of this recipe. Before trying any of the other recipes, we strongly encourage you to become comfortable with this recipe as it will help you understand the consistency we need to achieve with the dough when you try other bread recipes.

We use ordinary whole wheat bread with our basic recipe. This is a bread that is consistently available nationwide. And we had good success with our testers around the country.

Preparing this recipe requires a delicate balance. ④ Pureed foods are not a solid food you can pick up with your hands. And this recipe involves baking. It is easy to over-cook the ④ Pureed bread and it will be too firm. Rely on your test results to ensure proper preparation.

Avoid bread with lots of whole nuts and grains. They may NOT process properly to the smooth texture required for ④ Pureed. Although not required, we strongly suggest that you acquire some SimplyThick Bread Forms as they make the process very simple and easy. These are available at www.simplythick.com. Alternatively, you can use silicone egg rings for a pleasing presentation of pureed breads. Silicone egg rings are available at amazon.com.

INGREDIENTS

- 4 slices Honey Wheat or Whole Wheat Bread—look for a brand with about 70 calories per slice
- 3 oz. vegetable stock (if you are using a heavier or more dense bread, you may need another 1–2 oz. of vegetable stock)
- 2 tablespoons butter, softened or melted
- 1 egg
- 18g SimplyThick® EasyMix™— depending on the exact SimplyThick product(s) you have available to you this will be:
  - 3 strokes from a pump bottle or;
  - 3 ② Mildly Thick packets (6g)
- Pan release spray

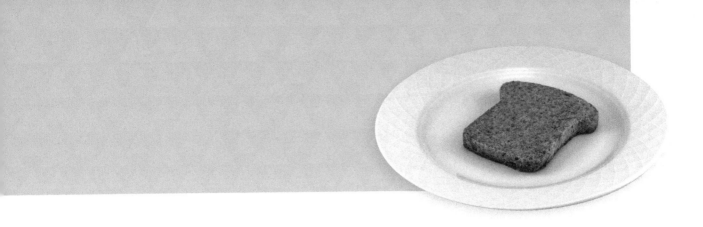

DIRECTIONS

1. Preheat the oven to 350° F.
2. Prepare cooking surfaces:
   a. If using 4 SimplyThick Bread Forms, spray each form with pan release spray and place on cookie sheet.
   b. If you don't have SimplyThick Bread Forms, you can use 4 silicone egg rings.
      i. Line baking sheet with parchment paper.
      ii. Place egg rings on parchment paper.
      iii. Spray with pan release spray.
3. Add the 4 slices of bread to a food processor with a sharp blade.
4. Put cover on processor.
5. Run processor until slices are processed into crumbs. This will usually only take about 5–10 seconds.
6. Add remaining ingredients—vegetable stock, butter, egg, and SimplyThick® EasyMix™.
7. Put cover on processor.
8. Run processor until all ingredients are thoroughly blended. Usually about 10–20 seconds.
9. Open the processor and inspect the contents of the processor bowl. Scrape sides and bottom of the processor bowl. Be sure there are no dry pieces of bread under the blade assembly.
10. Put cover on processor.
11. Run the processor until all lumps are eliminated, and there is a smooth texture. About 20–40 seconds.
12. If batter is too thick, add a little more vegetable stock, ½ oz. at a time and process thoroughly to achieve the correct batter texture.
13. Place batter in each of the 4 forms or rings prepared in Step 2.
14. Use a spatula to spread batter evenly in forms or rings. Avoid creating peaks in the batter.
15. Loosely cover with foil and place in oven.
16. Bake for 8–11 minutes to a minimum internal temperature of 160° F.
17. Let rest for 2 minutes after removing from oven.
18. Inspect for crusty outer edges and trim edges as needed.
19. Plate and serve, or store covered in the refrigerator for no more than 24 hours.
20. Evaluate to ensure compliance with IDDSI ④ Pureed requirements:
    a. No lumps and no separated water-thin liquids.
    b. Food sits on a mound above a dinner fork but does not drip or flow continuously through the fork.
    c. Easily separates and comes through the tines of a fork.
    d. Holds shape on a spoon, and slides off a teaspoon with little left—not sticky.

Toasted Whole Wheat Bread

NOTES

This is a variation of the basic ④ Pureed bread recipe. Before trying this recipe, we strongly encourage you to become comfortable with the basic ④ Pureed bread recipe so you understand what the correct batter texture looks like.

Toasting bread presents a couple of challenges to the process. First toasting does remove some moisture from the bread. Secondly, and more importantly, toasting can create really dry toasty bits that won't soften and can create bits that won't be appropriate for a true IDDSI ④ Pureed result. It is best to toast the bread lightly as this will give the flavor we are trying to add without introducing any other problems.

We use ordinary whole wheat bread with our basic recipe. This is a bread that is consistently available nationwide. And we had good success with our testers around the country.

Preparing this recipe requires a delicate balance. ④ Pureed foods are not a solid food you can pick up with your hands. And this recipe involves baking. It is easy to over-cook the ④ Pureed bread and it will be too firm. Rely on your test results to ensure proper preparation.

Avoid bread with lots of whole nuts and grains. They may NOT process properly to the smooth texture required for ④ Pureed. Although not required, we strongly suggest that you acquire some SimplyThick Bread Forms as they make the process very simple and easy. These are available at www.simplythick.com. Alternatively, you can use silicone egg rings for a pleasing presentation of pureed breads. Silicone egg rings are available at amazon.com.

INGREDIENTS

- 4 slices lightly toasted Honey Wheat or Whole Wheat Bread — look for a brand with about 70 calories per slice
- 3½ oz. vegetable stock (plus another ½–1 oz. on reserve, if needed)
- 2 tablespoons butter, softened or melted
- 1 egg
- 18g SimplyThick® EasyMix™— depending on the exact SimplyThick product(s) you have available to you this will be:
  - 3 strokes from a pump bottle or;
  - 3 ② Mildly Thick packets (6g)
- Pan release spray

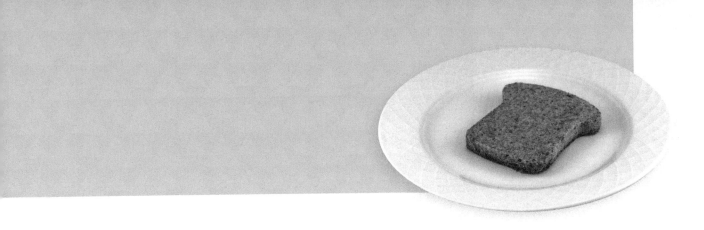

DIRECTIONS

1. Preheat the oven to 350° F.
2. Prepare cooking surfaces:
   a. If using 4 SimplyThick Bread Forms, spray each form with pan release spray and place on cookie sheet.
   b. If you don't have SimplyThick Bread Forms, you can use 4 silicone egg rings.
      i. Line baking sheet with parchment paper.
      ii. Place egg rings on parchment paper.
      iii. Spray with pan release spray.
3. Add the 4 slices of bread to a food processor with a sharp blade.
4. Put cover on processor.
5. Run processor until slices are processed into crumbs. This will usually only take about 5–10 seconds.
6. Add remaining ingredients—vegetable stock, butter, egg, and SimplyThick® EasyMix™.
7. Put cover on processor.
8. Run processor until all ingredients are thoroughly blended. Usually about 10–20 seconds.
9. Open the processor and inspect the contents of the processor bowl. Scrape sides and bottom of the processor bowl. Be sure there are no dry pieces of bread under the blade assembly.
10. Put cover on processor.
11. Run the processor until all lumps are eliminated, and there is a smooth texture. About 20–40 seconds.
12. If batter is too thick, add a little more vegetable stock, ½ oz. at a time and process thoroughly to achieve the correct batter texture.
13. Place batter in each of the 4 forms or rings prepared in Step 2.
14. Use a spatula to spread batter evenly in forms or rings. Avoid creating peaks in the batter.
15. Loosely cover with foil and place in oven.
16. Bake for 8–11 minutes to a minimum internal temperature of 160° F.
17. Let rest for 2 minutes after removing from oven.
18. Inspect for crusty outer edges and trim edges as needed.
19. Plate and serve, or store covered in the refrigerator for no more than 24 hours.
20. Evaluate to ensure compliance with IDDSI ▽4 Pureed requirements:
    a. No lumps and no separated water-thin liquids.
    b. Food sits on a mound above a dinner fork but does not drip or flow continuously through the fork.
    c. Easily separates and comes through the tines of a fork.
    d. Holds shape on a spoon, and slides off a teaspoon with little left—not sticky.

Toasted English Muffins

NOTES

This is a variation of the basic ▽④ Pureed bread recipe. Before trying this recipe, we strongly encourage you to become comfortable with the basic ▽④ Pureed bread recipe so you understand what the correct batter texture looks like.

Lightly toasted English muffins are required for this recipe to work properly. English muffins directly from their packaging tend to be too gummy to properly process. And while lightly toasting dries out the English muffin to allow it to properly process, darkly toasted English muffins may create toasty bits that are too dry to process to a true IDDSI ▽④ Pureed result. It is best to toast the muffins lightly as this will give the flavor and dryness we are trying to achieve without introducing the dry bits.

Preparing this recipe requires a delicate balance. ▽④ Pureed foods are not a solid food you can pick up with your hands. And this recipe involves baking. It is easy to over-cook the ▽④ Pureed bread and it will be too firm. Rely on your test results to ensure proper preparation.

Avoid English muffins with lots of whole nuts and grains. They may NOT process properly to the smooth texture required for ▽④ Pureed. Although not required, we strongly suggest that you acquire some SimplyThick Bread Forms as they make the process very simple and easy.

INGREDIENTS

- 2 English muffins, lightly toasted and cooled
- 3 oz. water (plus another ½–1 oz. on reserve, if needed)
- 2 tablespoons butter, softened or melted
- 1 egg
- 18g SimplyThick® EasyMix™— depending on the exact SimplyThick product(s) you have available to you this will be:
  - 3 strokes from a pump bottle or;
  - 3 ▲② Mildly Thick packets (6g)
- Pan release spray

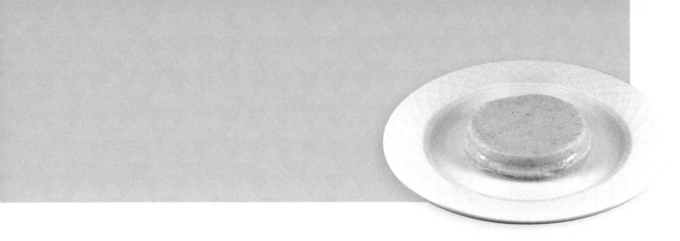

DIRECTIONS

1. Preheat the oven to 350° F.
2. Prepare cooking surfaces:
   a. If using 4 SimplyThick Bread Forms, spray each form with pan release spray and place on cookie sheet.
   b. If you don't have SimplyThick Bread Forms, you can use 4 silicone egg rings.
      i. Line baking sheet with parchment paper.
      ii. Place egg rings on parchment paper.
      iii. Spray with pan release spray.
3. Add the English muffins to a food processor with a sharp blade.
4. Put cover on processor.
5. Run processor until muffins are processed into crumbs. This will usually only take about 5–10 seconds.
6. Add remaining ingredients—water, butter, egg, and SimplyThick® EasyMix™.
7. Put cover on processor.
8. Run processor until all ingredients are thoroughly blended. Usually about 10–20 seconds.
9. Open the processor and inspect the contents of the processor bowl. Scrape sides and bottom of the processor bowl. Be sure there are no dry pieces of muffin under the blade assembly.
10. Put cover on processor.
11. Run the processor until all lumps are eliminated, and there is a smooth texture. About 20–40 seconds.
12. If batter is too thick, add a little more water, ½ oz. at a time and process thoroughly to achieve the correct batter texture.
13. Place batter in each of the 4 forms or rings prepared in Step 2.
14. Use a spatula to spread batter evenly in forms or rings. Avoid creating peaks in the batter.
15. Loosely cover with foil and place in oven.
16. Bake for 8–11 minutes to a minimum internal temperature of 160° F.
17. Let rest for 2 minutes after removing from oven.
18. Inspect for crusty outer edges and trim edges as needed.
19. Plate and serve, or store covered in the refrigerator for no more than 24 hours.
20. Evaluate to ensure compliance with IDDSI ④ Pureed requirements:
    a. No lumps and no separated water-thin liquids.
    b. Food sits on a mound above a dinner fork but does not drip or flow continuously through the fork.
    c. Easily separates and comes through the tines of a fork.
    d. Holds shape on a spoon, and slides off a teaspoon with little left—not sticky.

Cinnamon Raisin Bread

NOTES

This is a variation of the basic ④ Pureed bread recipe. Before trying this recipe, we strongly encourage you to become comfortable with the basic ④ Pureed bread recipe so you understand what the correct batter texture looks like.

Generally, we would prefer to use cinnamon bread without raisins, but it can be difficult to find. We have not had a problem when raisins are present in the bread, however it does mean you have to be on the lookout for unprocessed pieces.

Preparing this recipe requires a delicate balance. ④ Pureed foods are not a solid food you can pick up with your hands. And this recipe involves baking. It is easy to over-cook the ④ Pureed bread and it will be too firm. Rely on your test results to ensure proper preparation.

Avoid bread with lots of whole nuts and grains. They may NOT process properly to the smooth texture required for ④ Pureed. Although not required, we strongly suggest that you acquire some SimplyThick Bread Forms as they make the process very simple and easy.

INGREDIENTS

- 4 slices cinnamon raisin bread
- 3 oz. water (plus another ½–1 oz. on reserve, if needed)
- 2 tablespoons butter, softened or melted
- 1 egg
- 18g SimplyThick® EasyMix™— depending on the exact SimplyThick product(s) you have available to you this will be:
  - 3 strokes from a pump bottle or;
  - 3 ② Mildly Thick packets (6g)
- Pan release spray

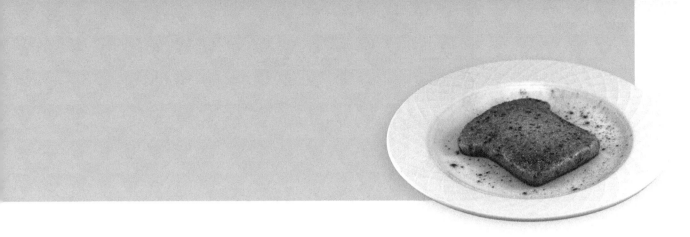

DIRECTIONS

1. Preheat the oven to 350° F.
2. Prepare cooking surfaces:
   a. If using 4 SimplyThick Bread Forms, spray each form with pan release spray and place on cookie sheet.
   b. If you don't have SimplyThick Bread Forms, you can use 4 silicone egg rings.
      i. Line baking sheet with parchment paper.
      ii. Place egg rings on parchment paper.
      iii. Spray with pan release spray.
3. Add the 4 slices of bread to a food processor with a sharp blade.
4. Put cover on processor.
5. Run processor until slices are processed into crumbs. This will usually only take about 5–10 seconds.
6. Add remaining ingredients—water, butter, egg, and SimplyThick® EasyMix™.
7. Put cover on processor.
8. Run processor until all ingredients are thoroughly blended. Usually about 10–20 seconds.
9. Open the processor and inspect the contents of the processor bowl. Scrape sides and bottom of the processor bowl. Be sure there are no dry pieces of bread under the blade assembly.
10. Put cover on processor.
11. Run the processor until all lumps are eliminated, and there is a smooth texture. About 20–40 seconds.
12. If batter is too thick, add a little more water, ½ oz. at a time and process thoroughly to achieve the correct batter texture.
13. Place batter in each of the 4 forms or rings prepared in Step 2.
14. Use a spatula to spread batter evenly in forms or rings. Avoid creating peaks in the batter.
15. Loosely cover with foil and place in oven.
16. Bake for 8–11 minutes to a minimum internal temperature of 160° F.
17. Let rest for 2 minutes after removing from oven.
18. Inspect for crusty outer edges and trim edges as needed.
19. Plate and serve, or store covered in the refrigerator for no more than 24 hours.
20. Evaluate to ensure compliance with IDDSI ④ Pureed requirements:
    a. No lumps and no separated water-thin liquids.
    b. Food sits on a mound above a dinner fork but does not drip or flow continuously through the fork.
    c. Easily separates and comes through the tines of a fork.
    d. Holds shape on a spoon, and slides off a teaspoon with little left—not sticky.

Toasted Cinnamon Raisin Bread

NOTES

This is a variation of the basic ④ Pureed bread recipe. Before trying this recipe, we strongly encourage you to become comfortable with the basic ④ Pureed bread recipe so you understand what the correct batter texture looks like.

Generally, we would prefer to use cinnamon bread without raisins, but it can be difficult to find. We have not had a problem when raisins are present in the bread, however it does mean you have to be on the lookout for unprocessed pieces.

Toasting bread presents a couple of challenges to the process. First toasting does remove some moisture from the bread. Secondly, and more importantly, toasting can create really dry toasty bits that won't soften and can create bits that won't be appropriate for a true IDDSI ④ Pureed result. It is best to toast the bread lightly as this will give the flavor we are trying to add without introducing any other problems.

Preparing this recipe requires a delicate balance. ④ Pureed foods are not a solid food you can pick up with your hands. And this recipe involves baking. It is easy to over-cook the ④ Pureed bread and it will be too firm. Rely on your test results to ensure proper preparation.

Avoid bread with lots of whole nuts and grains. They may NOT process properly to the smooth texture required for ④ Pureed. Although not required, we strongly suggest that you acquire some SimplyThick Bread Forms as they make the process very simple and easy.

INGREDIENTS

- 4 slices lightly toasted cinnamon raisin bread
- 3 oz. water (plus another ½–1 oz. on reserve, if needed)
- 2 tablespoons butter, softened or melted
- 1 egg
- 18g SimplyThick® EasyMix™— depending on the exact SimplyThick product(s) you have available to you this will be:
  – 3 strokes from a pump bottle or;
  – 3 ② Mildly Thick packets (6g)
- Pan release spray

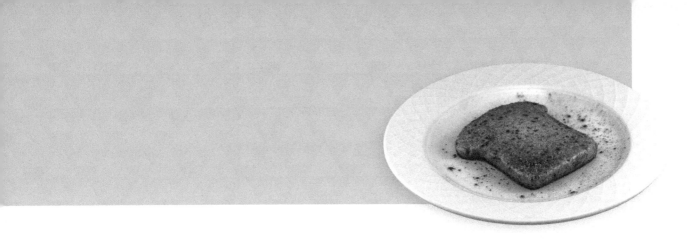

DIRECTIONS

1. Preheat the oven to 350° F.
2. Prepare cooking surfaces:
   a. If using 4 SimplyThick Bread Forms, spray each form with pan release spray and place on cookie sheet.
   b. If you don't have SimplyThick Bread Forms, you can use 4 silicone egg rings.
      i. Line baking sheet with parchment paper.
      ii. Place egg rings on parchment paper.
      iii. Spray with pan release spray.
3. Add the 4 slices of bread to a food processor with a sharp blade.
4. Put cover on processor.
5. Run processor until slices are processed into crumbs. This will usually only take about 5–10 seconds.
6. Add remaining ingredients—water, butter, egg, and SimplyThick® EasyMix™.
7. Put cover on processor.
8. Run processor until all ingredients are thoroughly blended. Usually about 10–20 seconds.
9. Open the processor and inspect the contents of the processor bowl. Scrape sides and bottom of the processor bowl. Be sure there are no dry pieces of bread under the blade assembly.
10. Put cover on processor.
11. Run the processor until all lumps are eliminated, and there is a smooth texture. About 20–40 seconds.
12. If batter is too thick, add a little more water, ½ oz. at a time and process thoroughly to achieve the correct batter texture.
13. Place batter in each of the 4 forms or rings prepared in Step 2.
14. Use a spatula to spread batter evenly in forms or rings. Avoid creating peaks in the batter.
15. Loosely cover with foil and place in oven.
16. Bake for 8–11 minutes to a minimum internal temperature of 160° F.
17. Let rest for 2 minutes after removing from oven.
18. Inspect for crusty outer edges and trim edges as needed.
19. Plate and serve, or store covered in the refrigerator for no more than 24 hours.
20. Evaluate to ensure compliance with IDDSI 4 Pureed requirements:
    a. No lumps and no separated water-thin liquids.
    b. Food sits on a mound above a dinner fork but does not drip or flow continuously through the fork.
    c. Easily separates and comes through the tines of a fork.
    d. Holds shape on a spoon, and slides off a teaspoon with little left—not sticky.

Refrigerated Cinnamon Rolls

NOTES

This is a variation of the basic ④ Pureed bread recipe. Before trying this recipe, we strongly encourage you to become comfortable with the basic ④ Pureed bread recipe so you understand what the correct batter texture looks like.

This recipe can be prepared using either 2 large or 4 small cinnamon rolls.

2 large cinnamon rolls—For this recipe, we start with the larger refrigerated cinnamon rolls cooked and cooled. These typically come with 5 rolls in a tube and are the larger rolls in the refrigerated dough section. Usually the package directions offer to cook these spread out on a cookie sheet or nestled in a cake pan. For our purposes, better results are usually achieved when cooked spread out on a cookie sheet.

4 small cinnamon rolls—For this recipe, we start with the classic refrigerated cinnamon rolls cooked and cooled. These typically come with 8 rolls in a tube and are the small ones.

The icing is probably best described as a Transitional Food within the IDDSI framework. If Transitional Foods are allowed in a person's diet, you can use the icing. Or skip it if needed.

Preparing this recipe requires a delicate balance. ④ Pureed foods are not a solid food you can pick up with your hands. And this recipe involves baking. It is easy to over-cook the ④ Pureed bread and it will be too firm. Rely on your test results to ensure proper preparation.

INGREDIENTS

- Cinnamon rolls
  - 2 large cooked and cooled refrigerated cinnamon rolls (Best results are achieved when these are cooked apart on a cookie sheet)

  or;
  - 4 small cooked and cooled refrigerated cinnamon rolls rolls (half a package of 8)
- 3 oz. water (plus another ½–1 oz. on reserve, if needed)
- 2 tablespoons butter, softened or melted
- 1 egg
- 18g SimplyThick® EasyMix™— depending on the exact SimplyThick product(s) you have available to you this will be:
  - 3 strokes from a pump bottle or;
  - 3 ▲ Mildly Thick packets (6g)
- Pan release spray

DIRECTIONS

1. Preheat the oven to 350° F.
2. Prepare cooking surfaces:
   a. If using 4 SimplyThick Bread Forms, spray each form with pan release spray and place on cookie sheet.
   b. If you don't have SimplyThick Bread Forms, you can use 4 silicone egg rings.
      i. Line baking sheet with parchment paper.
      ii. Place egg rings on parchment paper.
      iii. Spray with pan release spray.
3. Add the cinnamon rolls to a food processor with a sharp blade.
4. Put cover on processor.
5. Run processor until rolls are processed into crumbs. This will usually only take about 5–10 seconds.
6. Add remaining ingredients—water, butter, egg, and SimplyThick® EasyMix™.
7. Put cover on processor.
8. Run processor until all ingredients are thoroughly blended. Usually about 10–20 seconds.
9. Open the processor and inspect the contents of the processor bowl. Scrape sides and bottom of the processor bowl. Be sure there are no dry pieces of roll under the blade assembly.
10. Put cover on processor.
11. Run the processor until all lumps are eliminated, and there is a smooth texture. About 20–40 seconds.
12. If batter is too thick, add a little more water, ½ oz. at a time and process thoroughly to achieve the correct batter texture.
13. Place batter in each of the 4 forms or rings prepared in Step 2.
14. Use a spatula to spread batter evenly in forms or rings. Avoid creating peaks in the batter.
15. Loosely cover with foil and place in oven.
16. Bake for 8–11 minutes to a minimum internal temperature of 160° F.
17. Let rest for 2 minutes after removing from oven.
18. Inspect for crusty outer edges and trim edges as needed.
19. If allowed, spread icing on rolls.
20. Plate and serve, or store covered in the refrigerator for no more than 24 hours.
21. Evaluate to ensure compliance with IDDSI ▼4 Pureed requirements:
    a. No lumps and no separated water-thin liquids.
    b. Food sits on a mound above a dinner fork but does not drip or flow continuously through the fork.
    c. Easily separates and comes through the tines of a fork.
    d. Holds shape on a spoon, and slides off a teaspoon with little left—not sticky.

Pancakes From Mix

NOTES

This is a variation of the basic ④ Pureed bread recipe. Before trying this recipe, we strongly encourage you to become comfortable with the basic ④ Pureed bread recipe so you understand what the correct batter texture looks like.

Focus on using a basic, simple pancake mix. Any number of national boxed mixes will work. The key is to prepare the pancakes and let them cool completely before processing. If you don't cool the pancakes, they may be gummy in the processor. If you are in a hurry and can't wait to cool the pancakes, you can pulse them in the processor to break the pieces up. Then let cool for another 15 minutes.

Preparing this recipe requires a delicate balance. ④ Pureed foods are not a solid food you can pick up with your hands. And this recipe involves baking. It is easy to over-cook the ④ Pureed bread and it will be too firm. Rely on your test results to ensure proper preparation.

Remember to avoid mixes with lots of whole nuts and grains. They may NOT process properly to the smooth texture required for ④ Pureed.

INGREDIENTS

- Approximately 4.5 oz. prepared and cooled pancakes. This is about four 3½" pancakes
- 3½ oz. water (plus another ½–1 oz. on reserve, if needed)
- 2 tablespoons butter, softened or melted
- 1 egg
- 18g SimplyThick® EasyMix™— depending on the exact SimplyThick product(s) you have available to you this will be:
  - 3 strokes from a pump bottle or;
  - 3 ② Mildly Thick packets (6g)
- Pan release spray

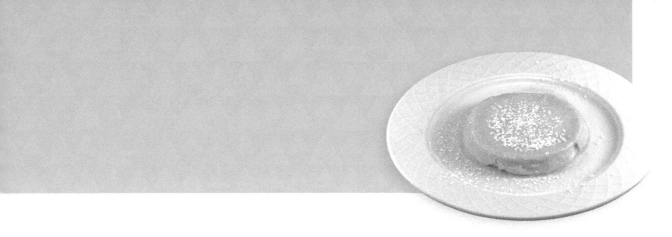

DIRECTIONS

1. Preheat the oven to 350° F.
2. Prepare cooking surfaces:
   a. If using 4 SimplyThick Bread Forms, spray each form with pan release spray and place on cookie sheet.
   b. If you don't have SimplyThick Bread Forms, you can use 4 silicone egg rings.
      i. Line baking sheet with parchment paper.
      ii. Place egg rings on parchment paper.
      iii. Spray with pan release spray.
3. Add the pancakes to a food processor with a sharp blade.
4. Put cover on processor.
5. Run processor until pancakes are processed into crumbs. This will usually only take about 5–10 seconds.
6. Add remaining ingredients—water, butter, egg, and SimplyThick® EasyMix™.
7. Put cover on processor.
8. Run processor until all ingredients are thoroughly blended. Usually about 10–20 seconds.
9. Open the processor and inspect the contents of the processor bowl. Scrape sides and bottom of the processor bowl. Be sure there are no dry pieces of pancake under the blade assembly.
10. Put cover on processor.
11. Run the processor until all lumps are eliminated, and there is a smooth texture. About 20–40 seconds.
12. If batter is too thick, add a little more water, ½ oz. at a time and process thoroughly to achieve the correct batter texture.
13. Place batter in each of the 4 forms or rings prepared in Step 2.
14. Use a spatula to spread batter evenly in forms or rings. Avoid creating peaks in the batter.
15. Loosely cover with foil and place in oven.
16. Bake for 8–11 minutes to a minimum internal temperature of 160° F.
17. Let rest for 2 minutes after removing from oven.
18. Inspect for crusty outer edges and trim edges as needed.
19. Plate and serve, or store covered in the refrigerator for no more than 24 hours.
20. Evaluate to ensure compliance with IDDSI ④ Pureed requirements:
    a. No lumps and no separated water-thin liquids.
    b. Food sits on a mound above a dinner fork but does not drip or flow continuously through the fork.
    c. Easily separates and comes through the tines of a fork.
    d. Holds shape on a spoon, and slides off a teaspoon with little left—not sticky.

Frozen Pancakes

NOTES

This is a variation of the basic ④ Pureed bread recipe. Before trying this recipe, we strongly encourage you to become comfortable with the basic ④ Pureed bread recipe so you understand what the correct batter texture looks like.

The key is to prepare the pancakes and let them cool completely before processing. If you don't cool the pancakes, they may be gummy in the processor. If you are in a hurry and can't wait to cool the pancakes, you can pulse them in the processor to break the pieces up. Then let cool for another 15 minutes.

Preparing this recipe requires a delicate balance. ④ Pureed foods are not a solid food you can pick up with your hands. And this recipe involves baking. It is easy to over-cook the ④ Pureed bread and it will be too firm. Rely on your test results to ensure proper preparation.

Remember to avoid pancakes with lots of whole nuts and grains. They may NOT process properly to the smooth texture required for ④ Pureed.

INGREDIENTS

- 1 serving frozen pancakes prepared and cooled. This is around three 4" pancakes, ⅞ oz. each
- 3 oz. water (plus another ½–1 oz. on reserve, if needed)
- 2 tablespoons butter, softened or melted
- 1 egg
- 18g SimplyThick® EasyMix™— depending on the exact SimplyThick product(s) you have available to you this will be:
  - 3 strokes from a pump bottle or;
  - 3 ② Mildly Thick packets (6g)
- Pan release spray

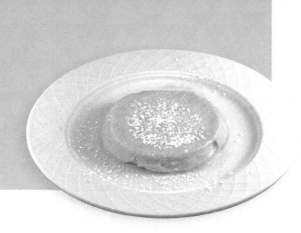

DIRECTIONS

1. Preheat the oven to 350° F.
2. Prepare cooking surfaces:
   a. If using 4 SimplyThick Bread Forms, spray each form with pan release spray and place on cookie sheet.
   b. If you don't have SimplyThick Bread Forms, you can use 4 silicone egg rings.
      i. Line baking sheet with parchment paper.
      ii. Place egg rings on parchment paper.
      iii. Spray with pan release spray.
3. Add the pancakes to a food processor with a sharp blade.
4. Put cover on processor.
5. Run processor until pancakes are processed into crumbs. This will usually only take about 5–10 seconds.
6. Add remaining ingredients—water, butter, egg, and SimplyThick® EasyMix™.
7. Put cover on processor.
8. Run processor until all ingredients are thoroughly blended. Usually about 10–20 seconds.
9. Open the processor and inspect the contents of the processor bowl. Scrape sides and bottom of the processor bowl. Be sure there are no dry pieces of pancake under the blade assembly.
10. Put cover on processor.
11. Run the processor until all lumps are eliminated, and there is a smooth texture. About 20–40 seconds.
12. If batter is too thick, add a little more water, ½ oz. at a time and process thoroughly to achieve the correct batter texture.
13. Place batter in each of the 4 forms or rings prepared in Step 2.
14. Use a spatula to spread batter evenly in forms or rings. Avoid creating peaks in the batter.
15. Loosely cover with foil and place in oven.
16. Bake for 8–11 minutes to a minimum internal temperature of 160° F.
17. Let rest for 2 minutes after removing from oven.
18. Inspect for crusty outer edges and trim edges as needed.
19. Plate and serve, or store covered in the refrigerator for no more than 24 hours.
20. Evaluate to ensure compliance with IDDSI ▽4 Pureed requirements:
    a. No lumps and no separated water-thin liquids.
    b. Food sits on a mound above a dinner fork but does not drip or flow continuously through the fork.
    c. Easily separates and comes through the tines of a fork.
    d. Holds shape on a spoon, and slides off a teaspoon with little left—not sticky.

Frozen Waffles

NOTES

This is a variation of the basic ⽥ Pureed bread recipe. Before trying this recipe, we strongly encourage you to become comfortable with the basic ⽥ Pureed bread recipe so you understand what the correct batter texture looks like.

The key is to prepare the waffles with very light browning in the toaster and to let them cool a little before processing. Toasting is doing two things for the waffle. It adds some flavor and removes some moisture. But with too much toasting, you can dry out the waffle too much and create really dry toasty bits that won't soften and can create bits that won't be appropriate for a true IDDSI ⽥ Pureed result. It is best to toast the waffles lightly as this will give the flavor we are trying to add without introducing any other problems.

Preparing this recipe requires a delicate balance. ⽥ Pureed foods are not a solid food you can pick up with your hands. And this recipe involves baking. It is easy to over-cook the ⽥ Pureed bread and it will be too firm. Rely on your test results to ensure proper preparation.

Remember to avoid waffles with lots of whole nuts and grains. They may NOT process properly to the smooth texture required for ⽥ Pureed.

INGREDIENTS

- 1 serving frozen waffles prepared and cooled. This is around three 3½" waffles, 1¼ oz. each
- 3½ oz. water (plus another ½–1 oz. on reserve, if needed)
- 2 tablespoons butter, softened or melted
- 1 egg
- 18g SimplyThick® EasyMix™—depending on the exact SimplyThick product(s) you have available to you this will be:
  – 3 strokes from a pump bottle or;
  – 3 ▲ Mildly Thick packets (6g)
- Pan release spray

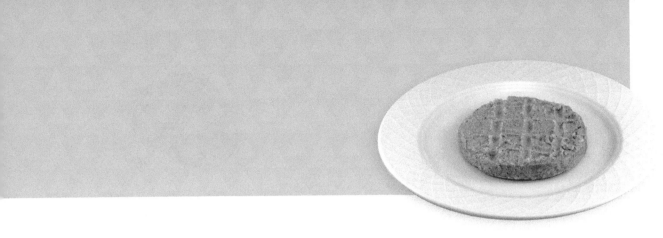

DIRECTIONS

1. Preheat the oven to 350° F.
2. Prepare cooking surfaces:
   a. If using 4 SimplyThick Bread Forms, spray each form with pan release spray and place on cookie sheet.
   b. If you don't have SimplyThick Bread Forms, you can use 4 silicone egg rings.
      i. Line baking sheet with parchment paper.
      ii. Place egg rings on parchment paper.
      iii. Spray with pan release spray.
3. Add the 3 waffles to a food processor with a sharp blade.
4. Put cover on processor.
5. Run processor until waffles are processed into crumbs. This will usually only take about 5–10 seconds.
6. Add remaining ingredients—water, butter, egg, and SimplyThick® EasyMix™.
7. Put cover on processor.
8. Run processor until all ingredients are thoroughly blended. Usually about 10–20 seconds.
9. Open the processor and inspect the contents of the processor bowl. Scrape sides and bottom of the processor bowl. Be sure there are no dry pieces of waffle under the blade assembly.
10. Put cover on processor.
11. Run the processor until all lumps are eliminated, and there is a smooth texture. About 20–40 seconds.
12. If batter is too thick, add a little more water, ½ oz. at a time and process thoroughly to achieve the correct batter texture.
13. Place batter in each of the 4 forms or rings prepared in Step 2.
14. Use a spatula to spread batter evenly in forms or rings. Avoid creating peaks in the batter.
15. Loosely cover with foil and place in oven.
16. Bake for 8–11 minutes to a minimum internal temperature of 160° F.
17. Let rest for 2 minutes after removing from oven.
18. Inspect for crusty outer edges and trim edges as needed.
19. Plate and serve, or store covered in the refrigerator for no more than 24 hours.
20. Evaluate to ensure compliance with IDDSI ▽④ Pureed requirements:
    a. No lumps and no separated water-thin liquids.
    b. Food sits on a mound above a dinner fork but does not drip or flow continuously through the fork.
    c. Easily separates and comes through the tines of a fork.
    d. Holds shape on a spoon, and slides off a teaspoon with little left—not sticky.

Beef (Steak or Roast)

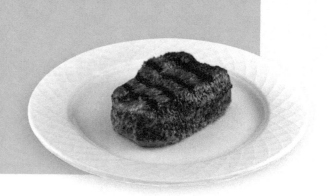

INGREDIENTS

- 16 oz. cooked and drained beef (hot or cold meat can be used—skin, bones, cartilage, gristle, excessive fat and crusty edges must be removed)
- ⚠ Extremely Thick Stock— see recipe on page 55

NOTES

Although this process works with both hot and cold meat, natural juices are released by hot meat, so less ⚠ Extremely Thick Stock will be needed when processing. On occasion with hot meat, no additional ⚠ Extremely Thick Stock may be needed to process properly. Rely on the process and your test results to ensure proper preparation.

DIRECTIONS

1. Add cooked beef into a food processor with sharp blade.
2. Put cover on processor.
3. Run processor for 15 seconds.
4. Open processor and inspect the contents of the processor bowl:
    a. Scrape sides and bottom of processor bowl.
    b. Remove any obviously undercooked, tough or stringy pieces.
    c. If any thin liquid begins to pool, drain or spoon out of processor.
5. Put cover on processor.
6. Start processor and add ⚠ Extremely Thick Stock to the processor about 1 oz. (approximately 2 tablespoons) at a time, until pureed consistency is achieved.
7. Using approximately 10 second intervals, process as long as necessary to eliminate all lumps:
    a. Stop the processor and scrape sides after each interval of processing.
    b. Typically, 2–3 rounds of processing and scraping will be needed.
8. Evaluate to ensure compliance with IDDSI ▼ Pureed requirements:
    a. No lumps and no separated water-thin liquids.
    b. Food sits on a mound above a dinner fork but does not drip or flow continuously through the fork.
    c. Easily separates and comes through the tines of a fork.
    d. Holds shape on a spoon, and slides off a teaspoon with little left—not sticky.
9. Remove from bowl and serve immediately, or separate into portions for storage in refrigerator or freezer.

Bonus presentation tip: Create the appearance of grill marks by "painting" on the puree with browning or barbecue sauce. We used Kitchen Bouquet® Browning & Seasoning Sauce in the photo above.

Ground Beef

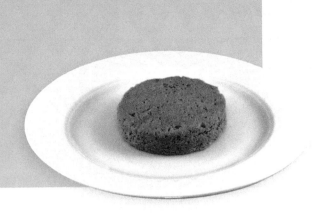

INGREDIENTS

- 16 oz. ground beef, cooked and drained of grease (hot or cold meat can be used—bones and gristle must be removed)
- 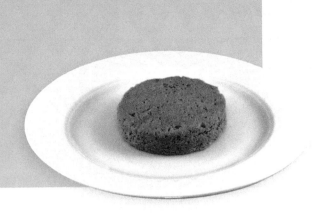 Extremely Thick Stock— see recipe on page 55

NOTES

Although this process works with both hot and cold meat, natural juices are released by hot meat, so less ⚠ Extremely Thick Stock will be needed when processing. On occasion with hot meat, no additional ⚠ Extremely Thick Stock may be needed to process properly. Rely on the process and your test results to ensure proper preparation.

DIRECTIONS

1. Add cooked ground beef to food processor with sharp blade.
2. Put cover on processor.
3. Run processor for 15 seconds.
4. Open processor and inspect the contents of the processor bowl:
   a. Scrape sides and bottom of processor bowl.
   b. Remove any obviously undercooked, tough or stringy pieces.
   c. If any thin liquid begins to pool, drain or spoon out of processor.
5. Put cover on processor.
6. Start processor and add ⚠ Extremely Thick Stock to the processor about ½ oz. at a time, until pureed consistency is achieved. We often found that less than 1 oz. of ⚠ Extremely Thick Stock was needed.
7. Using approximately 10 second intervals, process as long as necessary to eliminate all lumps:
   a. Stop the processor and scrape sides after each interval of processing.
   b. Typically, 2–3 rounds of processing and scraping will be needed.
8. Evaluate to ensure compliance with IDDSI ▽ Pureed requirements:
   a. No lumps and no separated water-thin liquids.
   b. Food sits on a mound above a dinner fork but does not drip or flow continuously through the fork.
   c. Easily separates and comes through the tines of a fork.
   d. Holds shape on a spoon, and slides off a teaspoon with little left—not sticky.
9. Remove from bowl and serve immediately, or separate into portions for storage in refrigerator or freezer.

Shredded Beef

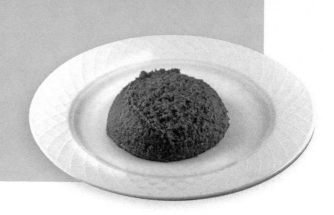

INGREDIENTS

- 16 oz. cooked shredded beef, drained of excess drippings (hot or cold meat can be used—skin, bones and cartilage must be removed)
- ⚠ Extremely Thick Stock— see recipe on page 55

NOTES

Although this process works with both hot and cold meat, natural juices are released by hot meat, so less ⚠ Extremely Thick Stock will be needed when processing. On occasion with hot meat, no additional ⚠ Extremely Thick Stock may be needed to process properly. Rely on the process and your test results to ensure proper preparation.

DIRECTIONS

1. Add shredded beef into food processor with sharp blade.
2. Put cover on processor.
3. Run processor for 15 seconds.
4. Open processor and inspect the contents of the processor bowl:
   a. Scrape sides and bottom of processor bowl.
   b. Remove any obviously undercooked, tough or stringy pieces.
   c. If any thin liquid begins to pool, drain or spoon out of processor.
5. Put cover on processor.
6. Start processor and add ⚠ Extremely Thick Stock to the processor about 1 oz. (approximately 2 tablespoons) at a time, until pureed consistency is achieved.
7. Using approximately 10 second intervals, process as long as necessary to eliminate all lumps:
   a. Stop the processor and scrape sides after each interval of processing.
   b. Typically, 2–3 rounds of processing and scraping will be needed.
8. Evaluate to ensure compliance with IDDSI ▽ Pureed requirements:
   a. No lumps and no separated water-thin liquids.
   b. Food sits on a mound above a dinner fork but does not drip or flow continuously through the fork.
   c. Easily separates and comes through the tines of a fork.
   d. Holds shape on a spoon, and slides off a teaspoon with little left—not sticky.
9. Remove from bowl and serve immediately, or separate into portions for storage in refrigerator or freezer.

PUREED

Meatloaf

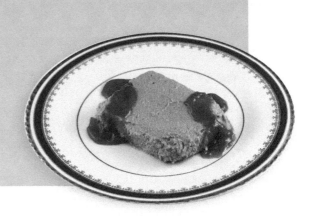

INGREDIENTS

- 13.2 oz. Stouffer's® Meatloaf or equivalent—microwaved per instructions
- Depending on end use, 4 oz. 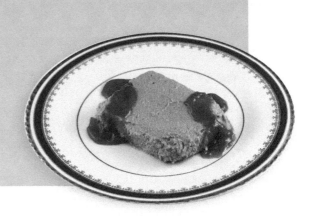 Extremely Thick Sauce or Stock— see Basic Sauce recipe on page 51 for ketchup glaze or BBQ sauce, or ④ Extremely Thick Stock recipe on page 55

NOTES

Since it is commonly available nationwide, most of our testing used Stouffer's® brand frozen meatloaf. Similar results were obtained with other frozen meatloaf brands. Other meatloaf brands may behave a little differently, however this recipe is designed to be flexible and allow you to ensure compliance with IDDSI guidelines.

This process will also work with homemade meatloaf.

DIRECTIONS

1. Drain any thin sauce or drippings and add cooked meatloaf to food processor with sharp blade.
2. Put cover on processor.
3. Run processor for 10 seconds.
4. Open processor and inspect meatloaf:
    a. Remove any obviously undercooked, tough or stringy pieces.
    b. Scrape all meat off the side of processor bowl.
    c. If any thin liquid begins to pool, drain or spoon out of processor.
5. Put cover on processor.
6. Start processor and if the meatloaf appears too dry or is clumping together, add ④ Extremely Thick Sauce or ④ Extremely Thick Stock, about 1 oz. at a time as needed, to achieve a pureed texture.
7. Using approximately 10 second intervals, process as long as necessary to eliminate all lumps:
    a. Remove cover and scrape sides after each interval of processing.
    b. Typically, 2–3 rounds of processing and scraping will be needed.
    c. If you cannot process to smooth, remove obvious lumps with a spoon.
8. Evaluate to ensure compliance with IDDSI ④ Pureed requirements:
    a. No lumps and no separated water-thin liquids.
    b. Food sits on a mound above a dinner fork but does not drip or flow continuously through the fork.
    c. Easily separates and comes through the tines of a fork.
    d. Holds shape on a spoon, and slides off a teaspoon with little left—not sticky.
9. Remove from bowl and serve immediately, or separate into portions for storage.

Meatballs

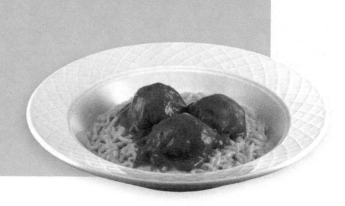

INGREDIENTS

- 12–16 oz. frozen or fresh made from scratch meatballs—cooked per package instructions
- Depending on end use, 4 oz. ④ Extremely Thick Sauce or Stock— see Marinara Sauce recipe on page 54, or ④ Extremely Thick Stock recipe on page 55

NOTES

These meatballs offer a flexible base for a variety of dishes. They can be used as a component of a pasta dish, a topping for ④ Pureed bread or simply covered with an appropriately thickened sauce. There are a variety of frozen meatballs available and each may behave a little differently, however this recipe is designed to be flexible and allow you to ensure compliance with IDDSI guidelines. This process will also work with homemade meatballs.

DIRECTIONS

1. Drain any thin sauce or drippings and add cooked meatballs to food processor with sharp blade.
2. Put cover on processor.
3. Run processor for 10 seconds.
4. Open processor and inspect meatballs:
   a. Remove any obviously undercooked, tough or stringy pieces
   b. Scrape all meat off the side of processor bowl.
   c. If any thin liquid begins to pool, drain or spoon out of processor.
5. Put cover on processor.
6. Start processor and add ④ Extremely Thick Sauce or ④ Extremely Thick Stock, about 1 oz. at a time as needed, to achieve a pureed texture.
7. Using approximately 10 second intervals, process as long as necessary to eliminate all lumps:
   a. Remove cover and scrape sides after each interval of processing.
   b. Typically, 2–3 rounds of processing and scraping will be needed.
   c. If you cannot process to smooth, remove obvious lumps with a spoon.
8. Evaluate to ensure compliance with IDDSI ④ Pureed requirements:
   a. No lumps and no separated water-thin liquids.
   b. Food sits on a mound above a dinner fork but does not drip or flow continuously through the fork.
   c. Easily separates and comes through the tines of a fork.
   d. Holds shape on a spoon, and slides off a teaspoon with little left—not sticky.
9. Remove from bowl in 1 oz. portions and form meatball shapes with clean sanitary hands or gloved hands. If meat is too soft to hold its shape, refrigerate for an hour and then roll into balls.
10. Add to final dish or store in refrigerator for later use.

Ham

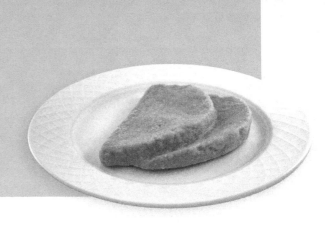

INGREDIENTS

- 16 oz. cooked ham, drained of excess drippings (hot or cold meat can be used—skin, bones and cartilage must be removed)
- ⚠ Extremely Thick Stock— see recipe on page 55

NOTES

We worked with convenience/ pre-packaged sliced or diced ham. Although this process works with both hot and cold meat, with the natural juices released by hot meat, less ⚠ Extremely Thick Stock will be needed when processing hot meat. On occasion with hot meat, no additional ⚠ Extremely Thick Stock may be needed to process properly. Rely on the process and your test results to ensure proper preparation.

DIRECTIONS

1. Add ham to food processor with sharp blade.
2. Put cover on processor.
3. Run processor for 15 seconds.
4. Open processor and inspect the contents of the processor bowl:
   a. Scrape sides and bottom of processor bowl.
   b. Remove any obviously undercooked, tough or stringy pieces.
   c. If any thin liquid begins to pool, drain or spoon out of processor.
5. Put cover on processor.
6. Start processor and add ⚠ Extremely Thick Stock to the processor about 1 oz. (approximately 2 tablespoons) at a time, until pureed consistency is achieved.
7. Using approximately 10 second intervals, process as long as necessary to eliminate all lumps:
   a. Stop the processor and scrape sides after each interval of processing.
   b. Typically, 2–3 rounds of processing and scraping will be needed.
8. Evaluate to ensure compliance with IDDSI ▽ Pureed requirements:
   a. No lumps and no separated water-thin liquids.
   b. Food sits on a mound above a dinner fork but does not drip or flow continuously through the fork.
   c. Easily separates and comes through the tines of a fork.
   d. Holds shape on a spoon, and slides off a teaspoon with little left—not sticky.
9. Remove from bowl and serve immediately, or separate into portions for storage in refrigerator or freezer.

Pulled Pork

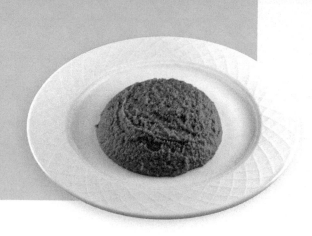

INGREDIENTS

- 16 oz. cooked pulled pork, drained of excess drippings (hot or cold meat can be used—skin, bones and cartilage must be removed)
- ④ Extremely Thick Stock— see recipe on page 55

NOTES

Although this process works with both hot and cold meat, natural juices are released by hot meat, so less ④ Extremely Thick Stock will be needed when processing. On occasion with hot meat, no additional ④ Extremely Thick Stock may be needed to process properly. Rely on the process and your test results to ensure proper preparation.

DIRECTIONS

1. Add pulled pork into food processor with sharp blade.
2. Put cover on processor.
3. Run processor for 15 seconds.
4. Open processor and inspect the contents of the processor bowl:
   a. Scrape sides and bottom of processor bowl.
   b. Remove any obviously undercooked, tough or stringy pieces.
   c. If any thin liquid begins to pool, drain or spoon out of processor.
5. Put cover on processor.
6. Start processor and add ④ Extremely Thick Stock to the processor about 1 oz. (approximately 2 tablespoons) at a time, until pureed consistency is achieved.
7. Using approximately 10 second intervals, process as long as necessary to eliminate all lumps:
   a. Stop the processor and scrape sides after each interval of processing.
   b. Typically, 2–3 rounds of processing and scraping will be needed.
8. Evaluate to ensure compliance with IDDSI ▽④ Pureed requirements:
   a. No lumps and no separated water-thin liquids.
   b. Food sits on a mound above a dinner fork but does not drip or flow continuously through the fork.
   c. Easily separates and comes through the tines of a fork.
   d. Holds shape on a spoon, and slides off a teaspoon with little left—not sticky.
9. Remove from bowl and serve immediately, or separate into portions for storage in refrigerator or freezer.

Pork Chops or Pork Loin

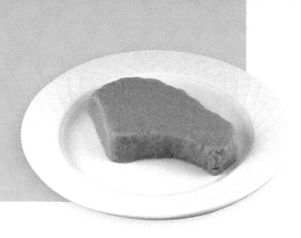

INGREDIENTS

- 16 oz. cooked pork chops or loin (hot or cold meat can be used—skin, bones and cartilage must be removed)
- 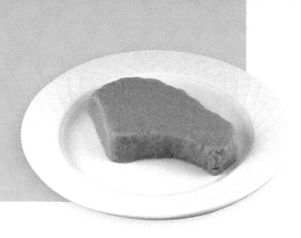 Extremely Thick Stock— see recipe on page 55

NOTES

Each batch of meat will process a little differently, so there is flexibility built into the recipe. Although this process works with both hot and cold meat, natural juices are released by hot meat, so less ▲ Extremely Thick Stock will be needed when processing. On occasion with hot meat, no additional ▲ Extremely Thick Stock may be needed to process properly. Rely on the process and your test results to ensure proper preparation.

DIRECTIONS

1. Add pork chops or pork loin to food processor with sharp blade.
2. Put cover on processor.
3. Run processor for 15 seconds.
4. Open processor and inspect the contents of the processor bowl:
    a. Scrape sides and bottom of processor bowl.
    b. Remove any obviously undercooked, tough or stringy pieces.
    c. If any thin liquid begins to pool, drain or spoon out of processor.
5. Put cover on processor.
6. Start processor and add ▲ Extremely Thick Stock to the processor about 1 oz. (approximately 2 tablespoons) at a time, until pureed consistency is achieved.
7. Using approximately 10 second intervals, process as long as necessary to eliminate all lumps:
    a. Stop the processor and scrape sides after each interval of processing.
    b. Typically, 2–3 rounds of processing and scraping will be needed.
    c. If you cannot process to smooth, remove obvious lumps with a spoon.
8. Evaluate to ensure compliance with IDDSI ▼ Pureed requirements:
    a. No lumps and no separated water-thin liquids.
    b. Food sits on a mound above a dinner fork but does not drip or flow continuously through the fork.
    c. Easily separates and comes through the tines of a fork.
    d. Holds shape on a spoon, and slides off a teaspoon with little left—not sticky.
9. Remove from bowl and serve immediately, or separate into portions for storage in refrigerator or freezer.

Chicken

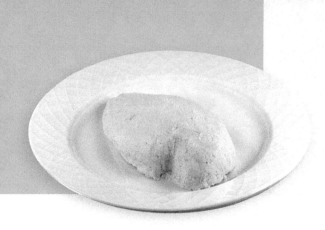

INGREDIENTS

- 16 oz. cooked and drained chicken (hot or cold meat can be used—skin, bones and cartilage must be removed)
- ⚠ Extremely Thick Stock— see recipe on page 55

NOTES

Although this process works with both hot and cold meat, natural juices are released by hot meat, so less ⚠ Extremely Thick Stock will be needed when processing. On occasion with hot meat, no additional ⚠ Extremely Thick Stock may be needed to process properly. Rely on the process and your test results to ensure proper preparation.

DIRECTIONS

1. Add cooked chicken to a food processor with sharp blade.
2. Put cover on processor.
3. Run processor for 15 seconds.
4. Open processor and inspect the contents of the processor bowl:
   a. Scrape sides and bottom of processor bowl.
   b. Remove any obviously undercooked, tough or stringy pieces.
   c. If any thin liquid begins to pool, drain or spoon out of processor.
5. Put cover on processor.
6. Start processor and add ⚠ Extremely Thick Stock to the processor about 1 oz. (approximately 2 tablespoons) at a time, until pureed consistency is achieved.
7. Using approximately 10 second intervals, process as long as necessary to eliminate all lumps:
   a. Stop the processor and scrape sides after each interval of processing.
   b. Typically, 2–3 rounds of processing and scraping will be needed.
8. Evaluate to ensure compliance with IDDSI ⚠ Pureed requirements:
   a. No lumps and no separated water-thin liquids.
   b. Food sits on a mound above a dinner fork but does not drip or flow continuously through the fork.
   c. Easily separates and comes through the tines of a fork.
   d. Holds shape on a spoon, and slides off a teaspoon with little left—not sticky.
9. Remove from bowl and serve immediately, or separate into portions for storage in refrigerator or freezer.

Bonus presentation tip: Use a food form—see page 34.

Boneless Buffalo Chicken Bites

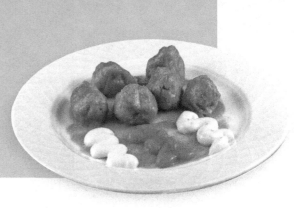

INGREDIENTS

- 12 oz. frozen fully cooked buffalo chicken breast strips
- ⚠ Extremely Thick Stock—see recipe on page 55*
- To taste or as desired:
  - Buffalo sauce thickened to ⚠ Extremely Thick—for more information see page 52
  - Ranch dressing thickened to ⚠ Extremely Thick—for more information see page 56
  - Blue Cheese dressing thickened to ⚠ Extremely Thick—for more information see page 57

NOTES

Each batch and brand of frozen chicken will behave a little differently and this recipe is designed to be flexible and allow you to ensure compliance with IDDSI guidelines.

DIRECTIONS

1. Heat frozen buffalo chicken breast strips in microwave oven or conventional oven according to instructions.
2. Add buffalo chicken breast to a food processor with sharp blade.
3. Put cover on processor.
4. Run processor for 15 seconds.
5. Open processor and inspect the contents of the processor bowl:
   a. Scrape sides and bottom of processor bowl.
   b. Remove any obviously undercooked, tough or stringy pieces.
   c. If any thin liquid begins to pool, drain or spoon out of processor.
6. Put cover on processor.
7. Start processor and add ⚠ Extremely Thick Stock to the processor about 1 oz. at a time, until ⚠ Pureed consistency is achieved. Generally, this will take 3–4 oz. of ⚠ Extremely Thick Stock for 12 oz. of chicken breast strips.
8. Using approximately 10 second intervals, process as long as necessary to eliminate all lumps:
   a. Stop the processor and scrape sides after each interval of processing.
   b. Typically, 2–3 rounds of processing and scraping will be needed.
9. Evaluate to ensure compliance with IDDSI ⚠ Pureed requirements:
   a. No lumps and no separated water-thin liquids.
   b. Food sits on a mound above a dinner fork but does not drip or flow continuously through the fork.
   c. Easily separates and comes through the tines of a fork.
   d. Holds shape on a spoon, and slides off a teaspoon with little left—not sticky.
10. Remove from food processor and roll ⚠ Pureed buffalo chicken into small irregular shapes to mimic "chicken bites."
11. Serve immediately or separate into portions for frozen storage.
12. When serving, if desired:
    a. Coat the "chicken bites" in ⚠ Extremely Thick Buffalo Sauce.
    b. Drizzle or spoon ⚠ Extremely Thick dressings—ranch and/or blue cheese—on plate for dipping.

On occasion, no ⚠ Extremely Thick Stock will be needed. But this could not be reproduced every time during our testing.

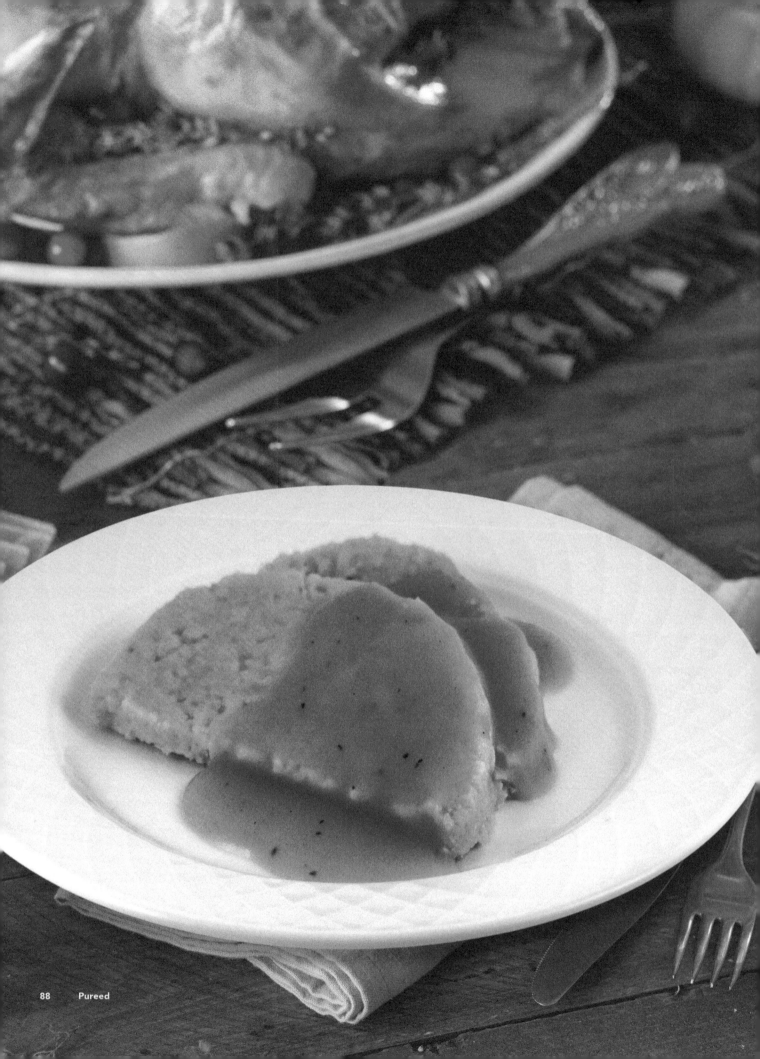

Turkey

INGREDIENTS

- 16 oz. cooked turkey meat (includes sandwich meat and other packaged and cooked turkey meat), drained of excess drippings (hot or cold meat can be used—skin and bones must be removed)
- ④ Extremely Thick Stock— see recipe on page 55

NOTES

Although this process works with both hot and cold meat, natural juices are released by hot meat, so less ④ Extremely Thick Stock will be needed when processing. On occasion with hot meat, no additional ④ Extremely Thick Stock may be needed to process properly. Rely on the process and your test results to ensure proper preparation.

DIRECTIONS

1. Add cooked turkey into food processor with sharp blade.
2. Put cover on processor.
3. Run processor for 15 seconds.
4. Open processor and inspect the contents of the processor bowl:
   a. Scrape sides and bottom of processor bowl.
   b. Remove any obviously undercooked, tough or stringy pieces.
   c. If any thin liquid begins to pool, drain or spoon out of processor.
5. Put cover on processor.
6. Start processor and add ④ Extremely Thick Stock to the processor about 1 oz. (approximately 2 tablespoons) at a time, until pureed consistency is achieved.
7. Using approximately 10 second intervals, process as long as necessary to eliminate all lumps:
   a. Stop the processor and scrape sides after each interval of processing.
   b. Typically, 2–3 rounds of processing and scraping will be needed.
8. Evaluate to ensure compliance with IDDSI ④ Pureed requirements:
   a. No lumps and no separated water-thin liquids.
   b. Food sits on a mound above a dinner fork but does not drip or flow continuously through the fork.
   c. Easily separates and comes through the tines of a fork.
   d. Holds shape on a spoon, and slides off a teaspoon with little left—not sticky.
9. Remove from bowl and serve immediately, or separate into portions for storage in refrigerator or freezer.

Breaded Fish or Fish Sticks

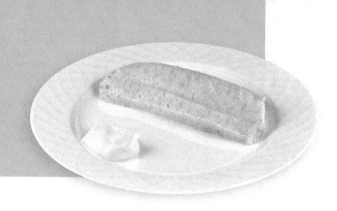

INGREDIENTS

- 16 oz. pre-cooked frozen "beer battered" cod fillets, or breaded fish sticks or equivalent—cooked according to the manufacturer's instructions and still warm or hot
- ▲4 Extremely Thick Stock— see recipe on page 55

NOTES

We DO NOT RECOMMEND storing portions of ▽4 Pureed breaded fish for later use. Our testers attempted to reheat portions of processed breaded fish that were stored in the refrigerator and freezer. The reheated stored portions were NOT able to pass IDDSI tests when reheated. The breading component became too sticky.

DIRECTIONS

1. Within 15 minutes of finishing cooking, add hot breaded fish to food processor with sharp blade. (Note: If breaded fish sits too long before processing, the breading will get gummy.)
2. Put cover on processor.
3. Run processor for 15 seconds.
4. Open processor and inspect the contents of the processor bowl:
   a. Scrape sides and bottom of processor bowl.
   b. Remove any obviously undercooked, tough or stringy pieces.
   c. If any thin liquid begins to pool, drain or spoon out of processor.
5. Put cover on processor.
6. Start processor and add ▲4 Extremely Thick Stock to the processor about 1 oz. (approximately 2 tablespoons) at a time, until pureed consistency is achieved.
7. Using approximately 10 second intervals, process as long as necessary to eliminate all lumps:
   a. Stop the processor and scrape sides after each interval of processing.
   b. Typically, 2–3 rounds of processing and scraping will be needed.
8. Evaluate to ensure compliance with IDDSI ▽4 Pureed requirements:
   a. No lumps and no separated water-thin liquids.
   b. Food sits on a mound above a dinner fork but does not drip or flow continuously through the fork.
   c. Easily separates and comes through the tines of a fork.
   d. Holds shape on a spoon, and slides off a teaspoon with little left—not sticky.
9. Remove from bowl and serve immediately. Do NOT store for later use.

Sauteed Fish

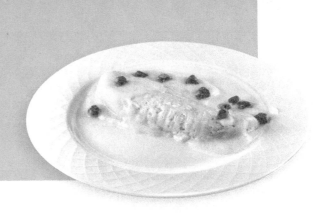

INGREDIENTS

- 16 oz. fish fillets, sauteed and "fork tender," drained of water-thin liquids (hot or cold meat can be used—skin and bones must be removed)
- 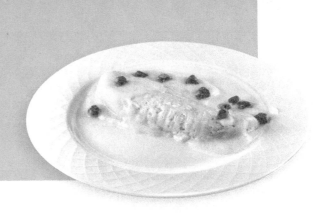 Extremely Thick Stock— see recipe on page 55

DIRECTIONS

1. Add sauteed fish to food processor with sharp blade.
2. Put cover on processor.
3. Run processor for 15 seconds.
4. Open processor and inspect the contents of the processor bowl:
   a. Scrape sides and bottom of processor bowl.
   b. Remove any obviously undercooked, tough or stringy pieces.
   c. If any thin liquid begins to pool, drain or spoon out of processor.
5. Put cover on processor.
6. Start processor and add ⚠ Extremely Thick Stock to the processor about 1 oz. (approximately 2 tablespoons) at a time, until pureed consistency is achieved.
7. Using approximately 10 second intervals, process as long as necessary to eliminate all lumps:
   a. Stop the processor and scrape sides after each interval of processing.
   b. Typically, 2–3 rounds of processing and scraping will be needed.
8. Evaluate to ensure compliance with IDDSI ⚠ Pureed requirements:
   a. No lumps and no separated water-thin liquids.
   b. Food sits on a mound above a dinner fork but does not drip or flow continuously through the fork.
   c. Easily separates and comes through the tines of a fork.
   d. Holds shape on a spoon, and slides off a teaspoon with little left—not sticky.
9. Remove from bowl and serve immediately, or separate into portions for storage in refrigerator or freezer.

Scrambled Eggs

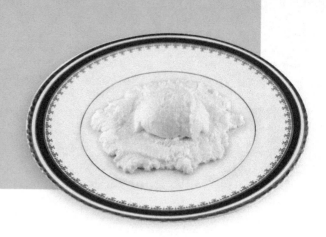

INGREDIENTS

- 4 eggs, scrambled and cooked (hot or cold)
- 2 oz. milk, slightly warmed to take the chill off
- 12g SimplyThick® EasyMix™— this is can be achieved with:
  - 2 strokes from a pump bottle or;
  - 2 ▲ Mildly Thick (6g) packets or;
  - 1 ⑧ Moderately Thick (12g) packet

NOTES

Unused portions can be frozen and re-heated to serve. Typically, you will not need to add more liquid to scrambled eggs to meet IDDSI standards. However, it is common for scrambled eggs to "give up" water-thin liquids. Be prepared to drain water-thin liquids and monitor closely while eating to avoid choking risk.

DIRECTIONS

1. Combine warm milk and SimplyThick® EasyMix™ in a small bowl and mix until well thickened—30–45 seconds. Set aside for Step 7.
2. Put eggs into food processor with sharp blade.
3. Put cover on processor.
4. Run processor for 5 seconds.
5. Open processor and inspect the contents of the processor bowl:
   a. Scrape sides and bottom of processor bowl.
   b. Remove any obviously burnt, overcooked, tough or stringy pieces.
   c. If any thin liquid begins to pool, drain or spoon out of processor.
6. Put cover on processor.
7. Start processor and add 1 oz. of thickened milk from Step 1.
8. Using approximately 10 second intervals, process as long as necessary to eliminate all lumps:
   a. Stop the processor and scrape sides after each interval of processing.
   b. Add more thickened milk from Step 1 if needed to control thin liquids or if desired for texture.
   c. Typically, 2–3 rounds of processing and scraping will be needed.
9. Evaluate to ensure compliance with IDDSI ④ Pureed requirements:
   a. No lumps and no separated water-thin liquids.
   b. Food sits on a mound above a dinner fork but does not drip or flow continuously through the fork.
   c. Easily separates and comes through the tines of a fork.
   d. Holds shape on a spoon, and slides off a teaspoon with little left—not sticky.
10. Remove from bowl and serve, or separate into portions for storage.

Bonus presentation tip: Photo shows a presentation when yolks and whites are separated, cooked, and processed separately.

Egg Salad

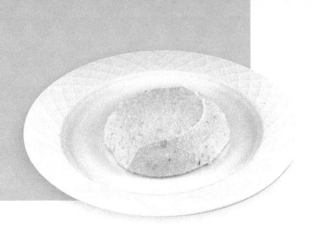

INGREDIENTS

- 16 oz. egg salad,* homemade or store-bought
- If necessary:
  – Mayonnaise

NOTES

We found that egg salad does not have ingredients that will be difficult to process. However, be on the lookout for celery, red and green peppers, or any nuts that would be difficult to process into a puree. Both celery and raw peppers are tough and fibrous and will not process into a smooth puree. Check the ingredient label to be certain. If you find an egg salad with these ingredients, it is easiest to manually remove them before processing. If you are following an egg salad recipe with these ingredients, simply omit them when you are making the egg salad. Egg salad may have red pimentos that look like red peppers, but these will process very easily.

DIRECTIONS

1. If any troublesome ingredients (as listed in the Notes on the left) are included on the label, add egg salad to a large mixing bowl. Remove any celery, red and green peppers, and any other obviously difficult to process pieces.
2. Add egg salad to food processor with a sharp blade.
3. Put cover on processor.
4. Run processor for 15 seconds.
5. Open processor and inspect the contents of the processor bowl:
   a. Scrape sides and bottom of processor bowl.
   b. Remove any obvious tough pieces (celery, peppers, nuts, etc.)
   c. If any thin liquid begins to pool, drain or spoon out of processor.
6. Put cover on processor.
7. Using approximately 10 second intervals, process as long as necessary to eliminate all lumps:
   a. Stop the processor and scrape sides after each interval of processing.
   b. Typically, 2–3 rounds of processing and scraping will be needed.
8. Evaluate to ensure compliance with IDDSI ④ Pureed requirements:
   a. No lumps and no separated water-thin liquids.
   b. Food sits on a mound above a dinner fork but does not drip or flow continuously through the fork.
   c. Easily separates and comes through the tines of a fork.
   d. Holds shape on a spoon, and slides off a teaspoon with little left—not sticky.
9. Remove from bowl and serve, or separate into portions for storage.

In our testing, we did not come across an egg salad that released water-thin liquids and we did not need to add any additional thick liquids to the egg salad when processed. If needed, add more mayonnaise to control any observed water-thin liquids.

Potato Salad

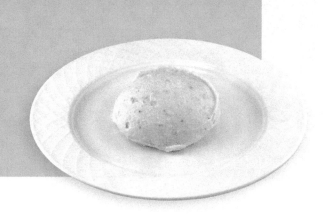

INGREDIENTS

- 16 oz. potato salad,*
  homemade or store-bought
- If necessary:
  – Mayonnaise

NOTES

We found that potato salad may not have ingredients that will be difficult to process. However, be on the lookout for celery, red and green peppers, or any nuts that would be difficult to process into a puree. Both celery and raw peppers are tough and fibrous and will not process into a smooth puree. Check the ingredient label to be certain. If you find a potato salad with these ingredients, it is easiest to manually remove them before processing. If you are following a potato salad recipe with these ingredients, simply omit them when you are making the potato salad.

DIRECTIONS

1. Add potato salad to a large mixing bowl. Remove any celery, red and green peppers, and any other obviously difficult to process pieces.
2. Add potato salad to food processor with a sharp blade.
3. Put cover on processor.
4. Run processor for 15 seconds.
5. Open processor and inspect the contents of the processor bowl:
   a. Scrape sides and bottom of processor bowl.
   b. Remove any obvious pieces of celery, peppers, nuts, or other tough pieces.
   c. If any thin liquid begins to pool, drain or spoon out of processor.
6. Put cover on processor.
7. Using approximately 10 second intervals, process as long as necessary to eliminate all lumps:
   a. Stop the processor and scrape sides after each interval of processing.
   b. Typically, 2–3 rounds of processing and scraping will be needed.
8. Evaluate to ensure compliance with IDDSI ④ Pureed requirements:
   a. No lumps and no separated water-thin liquids.
   b. Food sits on a mound above a dinner fork but does not drip or flow continuously through the fork.
   c. Easily separates and comes through the tines of a fork.
   d. Holds shape on a spoon, and slides off a teaspoon with little left—not sticky.
9. Remove from bowl and serve, or separate into portions for storage.

*In our testing, we did not come across a potato salad that released water-thin liquids and we did not need to add any additional thick liquids to the potato salad when processed. If needed, add more mayonnaise to control any observed water-thin liquids.

Chicken Salad

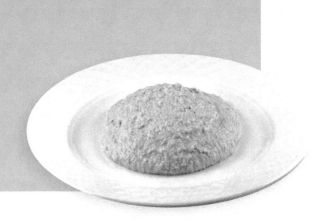

INGREDIENTS

- 16 oz chicken salad,*
  homemade or store-bought
- If necessary:
  – Mayonnaise

NOTES

We found wide variations in prepared chicken salad when our testers went shopping. Try to avoid products that have nuts, celery, peppers or similar ingredients that will be tough to process into a puree. Both celery and raw peppers are tough and fibrous and will not process into a smooth puree. Check the ingredient label to be certain. If you find a chicken salad with these ingredients, it is easiest to manually remove them before processing. If you are following a chicken salad recipe with these ingredients, simply omit them when you are making the chicken salad.

DIRECTIONS

1. Add chicken salad to a large mixing bowl. Remove any celery, nuts, red and green peppers and any other obviously difficult to process pieces.
2. Add chicken salad to food processor with a sharp blade.
3. Put cover on processor.
4. Run processor for 15 seconds.
5. Open processor and inspect the contents of the processor bowl:
   a. Scrape sides and bottom of processor bowl.
   b. Remove any obvious pieces of celery, peppers, nuts, or other tough pieces.
   c. If any thin liquid begins to pool, drain or spoon out of processor.
6. Put cover on processor.
7. Using approximately 10 second intervals, process as long as necessary to eliminate all lumps:
   a. Stop the processor and scrape sides after each interval of processing.
   b. Typically, 2–3 rounds of processing and scraping will be needed.
8. Evaluate to ensure compliance with IDDSI ▼ Pureed requirements:
   a. No lumps and no separated water-thin liquids.
   b. Food sits on a mound above a dinner fork but does not drip or flow continuously through the fork.
   c. Easily separates and comes through the tines of a fork.
   d. Holds shape on a spoon, and slides off a teaspoon with little left—not sticky.
9. Remove from bowl and serve, or separate into portions for storage.

In our testing, we did not come across a chicken salad that released water-thin liquids and we did not need to add any additional thick liquids to the chicken salad when processed. If needed, add more mayonnaise to control any observed water-thin liquids.

Tuna Salad

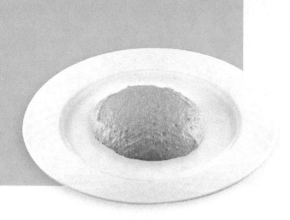

INGREDIENTS

- 16 oz. tuna salad,*
  homemade or store-bought
- If necessary:
  – Mayonnaise

NOTES

We found wide variations in prepared tuna salad when our testers went shopping. Try to avoid products that have pine nuts or similar ingredients that will be tough to process into a puree. Celery and red and green peppers are common ingredients in prepared tuna salad. Both celery and raw peppers are tough and fibrous and will not process into a smooth puree. They will have to be manually removed. If you make tuna salad from scratch, we recommend omitting peppers and celery from the recipe.

DIRECTIONS

1. Add tuna salad to a large mixing bowl. Remove any celery, red and green peppers and any other obviously difficult to process pieces.
2. Add tuna salad to food processor with a sharp blade.
3. Put cover on processor.
4. Run processor for 15 seconds.
5. Open processor and inspect the contents of the processor bowl:
   a. Scrape sides and bottom of processor bowl.
   b. Remove any obvious pieces of celery, peppers, nuts, or other tough pieces.
   c. If any thin liquid begins to pool, drain or spoon out of processor.
6. Put cover on processor.
7. Using approximately 10 second intervals, process as long as necessary to eliminate all lumps:
   a. Stop the processor and scrape sides after each interval of processing.
   b. Typically, 2–3 rounds of processing and scraping will be needed.
8. Evaluate to ensure compliance with IDDSI 4️ Pureed requirements:
   a. No lumps and no separated water-thin liquids.
   b. Food sits on a mound above a dinner fork but does not drip or flow continuously through the fork.
   c. Easily separates and comes through the tines of a fork.
   d. Holds shape on a spoon, and slides off a teaspoon with little left—not sticky.
9. Remove from bowl and serve, or separate into portions for storage.

*In our testing, we did not come across a tuna salad that released water-thin liquids and we did not need to add any additional thick liquids to the tuna salad when processed. If needed, add more mayonnaise to control any observed water-thin liquids.

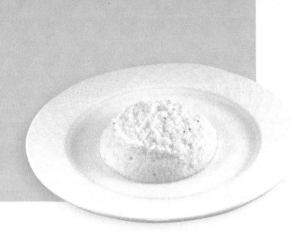

PUREED

Coleslaw

INGREDIENTS

- 16 oz. coleslaw, homemade or store-bought — drained of thin liquids
- 2–4 oz. mayonnaise, sour cream or 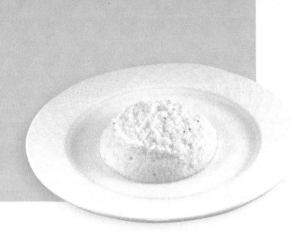 Extremely Thick Stock—see recipe on page 55

NOTES

There are variations in the ingredient list for prepared coleslaw. When shopping, try to avoid products that have celery, pickles, pine nuts, or similar ingredients that will be tough to process into a puree. If these are present and difficult to process, they will have to be manually removed. If you make coleslaw from scratch, we recommend avoiding difficult to process ingredients. Mayonnaise is our recommended Extremely Thick liquid to add to the coleslaw to turn it into a puree, but other Extremely Thick liquids will work as well. On occasion with coleslaw, no additional Extremely Thick liquid will be needed to process properly. Rely on the process and your test results to ensure proper preparation.

DIRECTIONS

1. Add coleslaw to a large mixing bowl. Remove any celery, red and green peppers, and any other obviously difficult to process pieces.
2. Add coleslaw to food processor with a sharp blade.
3. Put cover on processor.
4. Run processor for 15 seconds.
5. Open processor and inspect the contents of the processor bowl:
   a. Scrape sides and bottom of processor bowl.
   b. Remove any obvious pieces of celery, peppers, nuts, or other tough pieces.
   c. If any thin liquid begins to pool, drain or spoon out of processor.
6. Put cover on processor.
7. Using approximately 10 second intervals, process as long as necessary to eliminate all lumps:
   a. Stop the processor and scrape sides after each interval of processing.
   b. Typically, 2–3 rounds of processing and scraping will be needed.
8. Evaluate to ensure compliance with IDDSI Pureed requirements:
   a. No lumps and no separated water-thin liquids.
   b. Food sits on a mound above a dinner fork but does not drip or flow continuously through the fork.
   c. Easily separates and comes through the tines of a fork.
   d. Holds shape on a spoon, and slides off a teaspoon with little left—not sticky.
9. Remove from bowl and serve, or separate into portions for storage.

Mashed Potatoes

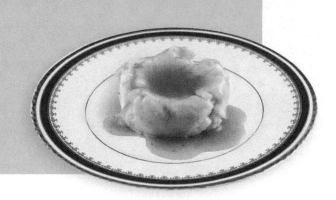

INGREDIENTS

- Potato flakes prepared according to package instructions—to yield 4 portions
- 2–4 tablespoons of butter, as needed
- ▲4 Extremely Thick Stock—see recipe on page 55

NOTES

Mashed potatoes are often used as the easiest example from our every day diet to explain what a ▽4 Pureed texture should be. However, when we offer this analogy, it is the whipped mashed potatoes—without skins, lumps, or cheese added—that is the texture and mouthfeel we are aiming for. Potatoes are very starchy and have the potential to become sticky—especially when they sit out. Adding additional butter relieves the stickiness inherent in potatoes.

Due to the simple and repeatable preparation, we have chosen to recommend using potatoes flakes in this book. If you want to make mashed potatoes from scratch, please keep 2 things in mind. First, eliminate the skins. We found it too difficult to process the skins into a nice lump-free ▽4 Pureed texture. And second, add extra butter to your recipe to keep the potatoes moist and soft for the 30 minutes we target with IDDSI compliant recipes.

Rely on the process and your test results to ensure proper preparation.

DIRECTIONS

1. Prepare potato flakes according to package instructions and put into mixing bowl.
2. Add 2 tablespoons butter and work vigorously into mashed potatoes until butter has been absorbed and is no longer visible. Add more butter to suit taste or as needed to reduce stickiness.
3. Evaluate to ensure compliance with IDDSI ▽4 Pureed requirements:
   a. No lumps and no separated water-thin liquids.
   b. Food sits on a mound above a dinner fork but does not drip or flow continuously through the fork.
   c. Easily separates and comes through the tines of a fork.
   d. Holds shape on a spoon, and slides off a teaspoon with little left—not sticky.
4. If mashed potatoes are too sticky, return to Step 2.
5. Remove from mixing bowl and serve, or separate into portions for storage.

Bonus presentation tip: Put ▽4 Pureed mashed potatoes into a pastry bag with tip, or zip-style plastic bag. Use pastry tip or cut off corner of bag to pipe pureed potatoes onto plate for improved presentation.

Carrots

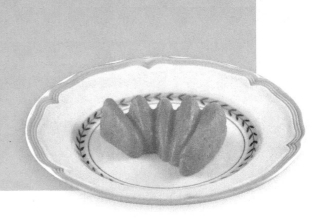

INGREDIENTS

- 2 cups (16 oz.) carrots cooked until tender enough to be pierced or cut easily with a fork (hot or cold)
- 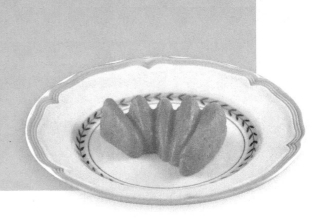 Extremely Thick Stock— see recipe on page 55

NOTES

This process will work with both hot and cold cooked carrots. The total amount of Extremely Thick Stock needed will vary based on whether you start with canned, frozen, or fresh carrots. Canned carrots, even after draining, will carry more liquid with them into the food processor than the fresh or frozen carrots. On occasion, you may find that no additional Extremely Thick Stock is required to process properly. Rely on the process and your test results to ensure proper preparation.

DIRECTIONS

1. Add cooked carrots to food processor with sharp blade.
2. Put cover on processor.
3. Run processor for 15 seconds.
4. Open processor and inspect the contents of the processor bowl:
    a. Scrape sides and bottom of processor bowl.
    b. Remove any obviously undercooked, tough or stringy pieces.
    c. If thin liquid begins to pool, drain or spoon out of processor.
5. Put cover on processor.
6. Start processor and add Extremely Thick Stock to the processor about 1 oz. (approximately 2 tablespoons) at a time, until pureed consistency is achieved.
7. Using approximately 10 second intervals, process as long as necessary to eliminate all lumps:
    a. Stop the processor and scrape sides after each interval of processing.
    b. Typically, 2–3 rounds of processing and scraping will be needed.
    c. If you cannot process to smooth, remove obvious lumps with a spoon.
8. Evaluate to ensure compliance with IDDSI Pureed requirements:
    a. No lumps and no separated water-thin liquids.
    b. Food sits on a mound above a dinner fork but does not drip or flow continuously through the fork.
    c. Easily separates and comes through the tines of a fork.
    d. Holds shape on a spoon, and slides off a teaspoon with little left—not sticky.
9. Remove from bowl and serve immediately, or separate into portions for storage in refrigerator or freezer.

Bonus presentation tip: Put Pureed Carrots into a pastry bag with tip, or zip-style plastic bag. Use pastry tip or cut off corner of bag to pipe onto plate for improved presentation.

Cauliflower

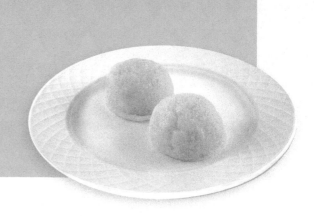

INGREDIENTS

- 2 cups (16 oz.) cauliflower cooked until tender enough to be pierced or cut easily with a fork (hot or cold)
- 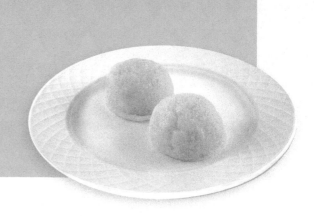 Extremely Thick Stock— see recipe on page 55

NOTES

This process will work with both hot and cold cooked cauliflower. The total amount of ⚠ Extremely Thick Stock needed will vary based on whether you start with frozen or fresh cauliflower, and whether you cook it in the microwave or by steaming. Cooking cauliflower to well done will reduce the processing time. With cauliflower, you may find that no additional ⚠ Extremely Thick Stock is required to process properly. Rely on the process and your test results to ensure proper preparation.

DIRECTIONS

1. Add cooked cauliflower to food processor with sharp blade.
2. Put cover on processor.
3. Run processor for 15 seconds.
4. Open processor and inspect the contents of the processor bowl:
   a. Scrape sides and bottom of processor bowl.
   b. Remove any obviously undercooked, tough or stringy pieces.
   c. If thin liquid begins to pool, drain or spoon out of processor.
5. Put cover on processor.
6. Start processor and add ⚠ Extremely Thick Stock to the processor about 1 oz. (approximately 2 tablespoons) at a time, until pureed consistency is achieved.
7. Using approximately 10 second intervals, process as long as necessary to eliminate all lumps:
   a. Stop the processor and scrape sides after each interval of processing.
   b. Typically, 2–3 rounds of processing and scraping will be needed.
   c. If you cannot process to smooth, remove obvious lumps with a spoon.
8. Evaluate to ensure compliance with IDDSI ▽ Pureed requirements:
   a. No lumps and no separated water-thin liquids.
   b. Food sits on a mound above a dinner fork but does not drip or flow continuously through the fork.
   c. Easily separates and comes through the tines of a fork.
   d. Holds shape on a spoon, and slides off a teaspoon with little left—not sticky.
9. Remove from bowl and serve immediately, or separate into portions for storage in refrigerator or freezer.

Bonus presentation tip: Put ▽ Pureed Cauliflower into a pastry bag with tip, or zip-style plastic bag. Use pastry tip or cut off corner of bag to pipe onto plate for improved presentation.

Broccoli

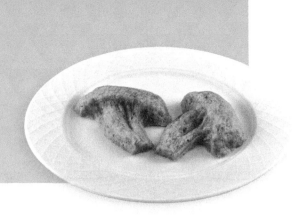

INGREDIENTS

- 2 cups (16 oz.) broccoli cooked until the thicker stems are tender enough to be pierced or cut easily with a fork (hot or cold)
- 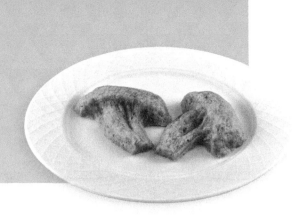 Extremely Thick Stock— see recipe on page 55

NOTES

This process will work with both hot and cold cooked broccoli. The total amount of ▲ Extremely Thick stock needed will vary based on whether you start with frozen or fresh broccoli, and whether you cook in the microwave or by steaming. Rely on the process and your test results to ensure proper preparation.

DIRECTIONS

1. Add cooked broccoli to food processor with sharp blade.
2. Put cover on processor.
3. Run processor for 15 seconds.
4. Open processor and inspect the contents of the processor bowl:
    a. Scrape sides and bottom of processor bowl.
    b. Remove any obviously undercooked, tough or stringy pieces.
    c. Watch for and remove any particularly stiff, firm stems that are not processing easily.
    d. If any thin liquid begins to pool, drain or spoon out of processor.
5. Put cover on processor.
6. Start processor and add ▲ Extremely Thick Stock to the processor about 1 oz. (approximately 2 tablespoons) at a time, until pureed consistency is achieved.
7. Using approximately 10 second intervals, process as long as necessary to eliminate all lumps:
    a. Stop the processor and scrape sides after each interval of processing.
    b. Typically, 2–3 rounds of processing and scraping will be needed.
    c. If you cannot process to smooth, remove obvious lumps with a spoon.
8. Evaluate to ensure compliance with IDDSI ▲ Pureed requirements:
    a. No lumps and no separated water-thin liquids.
    b. Food sits on a mound above a dinner fork but does not drip or flow continuously through the fork.
    c. Easily separates and comes through the tines of a fork.
    d. Holds shape on a spoon, and slides off a teaspoon with little left—not sticky.
9. Remove from bowl and serve immediately, or separate into portions for storage in refrigerator or freezer.

Bonus presentation tip: Put ▲ Pureed Broccoli into a pastry bag with tip, or zip-style plastic bag. Use pastry tip or cut off corner of bag to pipe onto plate for improved presentation.

Butternut Squash

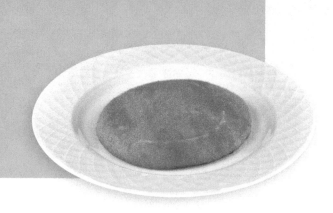

INGREDIENTS

- 2 cups (16 oz.) butternut squash (hot or cold) cooked until tender enough to be pierced or cut easily with a fork and drained thoroughly
- △ Extremely Thick Stock— see recipe on page 55

NOTES

This process will work with both hot and cold cooked butternut squash. The ripeness, moistness and softness of the particular butternut squash you are processing will impact the amount of △ Extremely Thick Stock needed to hold the puree together. With some butternut squashes, you may find that no additional △ Extremely Thick Stock is required to process properly. Rely on the process and your test results to ensure proper preparation.

DIRECTIONS

1. Add cooked butternut squash to food processor with sharp blade.
2. Put cover on processor.
3. Run processor for 15 seconds.
4. Open processor and inspect the contents of the processor bowl:
   a. Scrape sides and bottom of processor bowl.
   b. Remove any obviously undercooked, tough or stringy pieces.
   c. If thin liquid begins to pool, drain or spoon out of processor.
5. Put cover on processor.
6. Start processor and add △ Extremely Thick Stock to the processor about 1 oz. (approximately 2 tablespoons) at a time, until pureed consistency is achieved.
7. Using approximately 10 second intervals, process as long as necessary to eliminate all lumps:
   a. Stop the processor and scrape sides after each interval of processing.
   b. Typically, 2–3 rounds of processing and scraping will be needed.
   c. If you cannot process to smooth, remove obvious lumps with a spoon.
8. Evaluate to ensure compliance with IDDSI ▽ Pureed requirements:
   a. No lumps and no separated water-thin liquids.
   b. Food sits on a mound above a dinner fork but does not drip or flow continuously through the fork.
   c. Easily separates and comes through the tines of a fork.
   d. Holds shape on a spoon, and slides off a teaspoon with little left—not sticky.
9. Remove from bowl and serve immediately or separate into portions for storage in refrigerator or freezer.

Bonus presentation tip: Put ▽ Pureed Butternut Squash into a pastry bag with tip, or zip-style plastic bag. Use pastry tip or cut off corner of bag to pipe onto plate for improved presentation.

PUREED

Green Beans

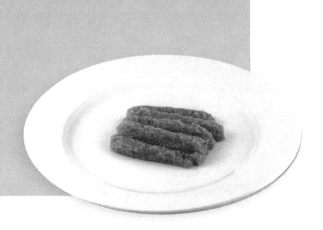

INGREDIENTS

- 2 cups (16 oz.) green beans cooked until tender enough to be pierced or cut easily with a fork, drained of all drippings and thin liquids (hot or cold)
- 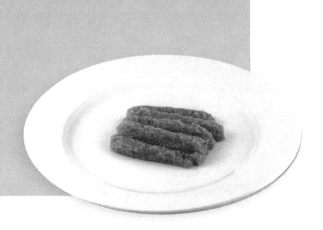 Extremely Thick Stock— see recipe on page 55

NOTES

This process will work with both hot and cold cooked green beans. The amount of Extremely Thick Stock needed will vary based on whether you are using canned, frozen, or fresh green beans. Even after draining, canned beans brought significantly more thin liquid into the food processor and required more Extremely Thick Stock. However, you may find that no additional Extremely Thick Stock is required to process properly into a perfect puree. Rely on the process and your test results to ensure proper preparation.

DIRECTIONS

1. Add cooked green beans to a food processor with sharp blade.
2. Put cover on processor.
3. Run processor for 15 seconds.
4. Open processor and inspect the contents of the processor bowl:
   a. Scrape sides and bottom of processor bowl.
   b. Remove any obviously undercooked, tough or stringy pieces.
   c. If thin liquid begins to pool, drain or spoon out of processor.
5. Put cover on processor.
6. Start processor and add Extremely Thick Stock to the processor about 1 oz. (approximately 2 tablespoons) at a time, until pureed consistency is achieved.
7. Using approximately 10 second intervals, process as long as necessary to eliminate all lumps:
   a. Stop the processor and scrape sides after each interval of processing.
   b. Typically, 2–3 rounds of processing and scraping will be needed.
   c. If you cannot process to smooth, remove obvious lumps with a spoon.
8. Evaluate to ensure compliance with IDDSI Pureed requirements:
   a. No lumps and no separated water-thin liquids.
   b. Food sits on a mound above a dinner fork but does not drip or flow continuously through the fork.
   c. Easily separates and comes through the tines of a fork.
   d. Holds shape on a spoon, and slides off a teaspoon with little left—not sticky.
9. Remove from bowl and serve immediately, or separate into portions for storage in refrigerator or freezer.

Bonus presentation tip: Add a 10.5 oz can of condensed cream of mushroom soup to a blender or food processor. Run until smooth. Heat and spoon on top of pureed beans for a green bean casserole presentation and flavor. In our testing, the condensed cream of mushroom soup did NOT require any Extremely Thick Stock or other thickener to meet IDDSI guidelines for Pureed.

Peas

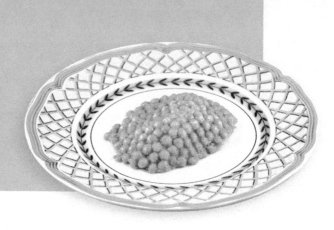

INGREDIENTS

- 2 cups (16 oz.) peas cooked until tender enough to be pierced or cut easily with a fork and drained thoroughly (hot or cold)
- ⚠ Extremely Thick Stock— see recipe on page 55

NOTES

This process will work with both hot and cold cooked peas.* The total amount of ⚠ Extremely Thick Stock needed will be influenced by the packaging of the peas—canned, frozen, or fresh—and the method of cooking—microwave or steaming. Canned peas will bring more liquid with them into the food processor than fresh or frozen peas. Depending on these factors, you may find it is NOT necessary to add ⚠ Extremely Thick Stock to process properly. Rely on the process and your test results to ensure proper preparation.

DIRECTIONS

1. Add cooked peas into food processor with sharp blade.
2. Put cover on processor.
3. Run processor for 15 seconds.
4. Open processor and inspect the contents of the processor bowl:
   a. Scrape sides and bottom of processor bowl.
   b. Remove any obviously undercooked, tough or stringy pieces or skins.
   c. If thin liquid begins to pool, drain or spoon out of processor.
5. Put cover on processor.
6. Start processor and add ⚠ Extremely Thick Stock to the processor about 1 oz. at a time, as needed until pureed consistency is achieved.
7. Using approximately 10 second intervals, process as long as necessary to eliminate all lumps:
   a. Stop the processor and scrape sides after each interval of processing.
   b. Typically, 2–3 rounds of processing and scraping will be needed.
   c. If you cannot process to smooth, remove obvious lumps with a spoon.
8. Evaluate to ensure compliance with IDDSI ④ Pureed requirements:
   a. No lumps and no separated water-thin liquids.
   b. Food sits on a mound above a dinner fork but does not drip or flow continuously through the fork.
   c. Easily separates and comes through the tines of a fork.
   d. Holds shape on a spoon, and slides off a teaspoon with little left—not sticky.
9. Remove from bowl and serve immediately, or separate into portions for storage in refrigerator or freezer.

Bonus presentation tip: Put ④ Pureed Peas into a pastry bag with tip, or zip-style plastic bag. Use pastry tip or cut off corner of bag to pipe onto plate for improved presentation.

*Warning: The skin or hull of a pea can pose a particular challenge when trying to modify the texture. Depending on the ripeness, manufacturing & packaging processes, and cooking techniques, the skin could still be too tough to pass the IDDSI ④ Pureed requirements. Use extra caution when working with peas to ensure any tough skin does not make it into the final product.

Spinach

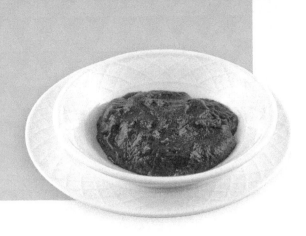

INGREDIENTS

- 2 cups (16 oz.) spinach cooked until tender enough to be cut easily with a fork, drained thoroughly (hot or cold)
- 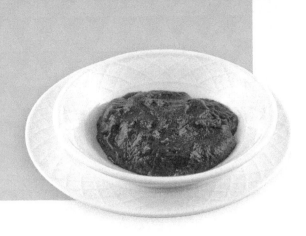 Extremely Thick Stock— see recipe on page 55

NOTES

This process will work with both hot and cold cooked spinach.* The amount of 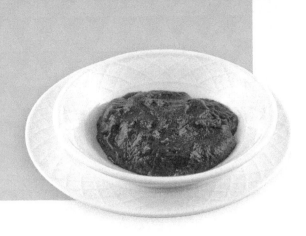 Extremely Thick Stock will vary depending on whether you are using canned, frozen, or fresh cooked spinach. You may find that no additional 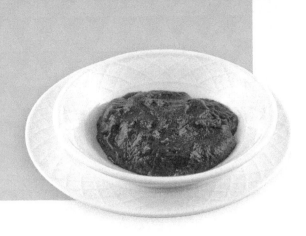 Extremely Thick Stock is required to process properly. Rely on the process and your test results to ensure proper preparation.

DIRECTIONS

1. Add cooked spinach to food processor with sharp blade.
2. Put cover on processor.
3. Run processor for 15 seconds.
4. Open processor and inspect the contents of the processor bowl:
    a. Scrape sides and bottom of processor bowl.
    b. Remove any obviously undercooked, tough or stringy pieces or stems.
    c. If thin liquid begins to pool, drain or spoon out of processor.
5. Put cover on processor.
6. Start processor and add 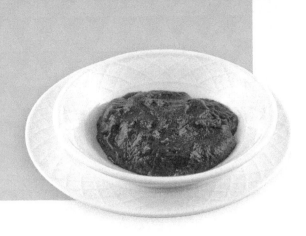 Extremely Thick Stock to the processor about 1 oz. at a time, as needed until pureed consistency is achieved.
7. Using approximately 10 second intervals, process as long as necessary to eliminate all lumps:
    a. Stop the processor and scrape sides after each interval of processing.
    b. Typically, 2–3 rounds of processing and scraping will be needed.
    c. If you cannot process to smooth, remove obvious lumps with a spoon.
8. Evaluate to ensure compliance with IDDSI 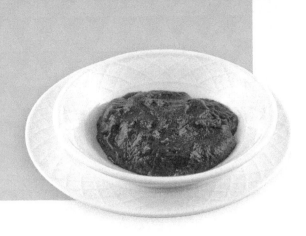 Pureed requirements:
    a. No lumps and no separated water-thin liquids.
    b. Food sits on a mound above a dinner fork but does not drip or flow continuously through the fork.
    c. Easily separates and comes through the tines of a fork.
    d. Holds shape on a spoon, and slides off a teaspoon with little left—not sticky.
9. Remove from bowl and serve immediately, or separate into portions for storage in refrigerator or freezer.

Bonus presentation tip: Put 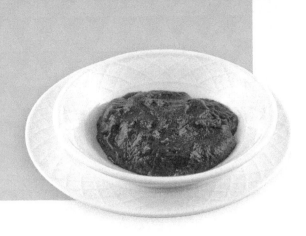 Pureed Cooked Spinach into a pastry bag with tip or zip-style plastic bag. Use a pastry tip or cut off a corner of the bag to pipe onto plate for improved presentation.

*Warning: The stems of spinach — especially fresh baby spinach — can pose a particular challenge to successfully puree. Many factors such as the ripeness, manufacturing process, packaging processes, and even cooking techniques, can leave the stems difficult to puree thoroughly. Use extra caution when working with cooked spinach to ensure tough stems do not make it into the final product.

Peaches

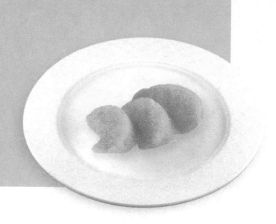

INGREDIENTS

- 16 oz. of peaches—thawed, peeled, rinsed and drained, as appropriate
- ⚠ Extremely Thick Stock— see recipe on page 55

NOTES

The total amount of ⚠ Extremely Thick Stock needed will vary on whether you start with canned, frozen, or fresh peaches. Canned peaches will carry more liquid with them into the food processor than the fresh or frozen peaches. Frozen peaches should be warmed before processing. Fresh peaches should be ripe and soft. On occasion, you may find that no additional ⚠ Extremely Thick Stock is required to process properly. Rely on the process and your test results to ensure proper preparation.

DIRECTIONS

1. Add peaches to food processor with sharp blade.
2. Put cover on processor.
3. Run processor for 15 seconds.
4. Open processor and inspect the contents of the processor bowl:
    a. Scrape sides and bottom of processor bowl.
    b. Remove any obviously tough or stringy pieces.
    c. If thin liquid begins to pool, drain or spoon out of processor.
5. Put cover on processor.
6. Start processor and add ⚠ Extremely Thick Stock to the processor about 1 oz. (approximately 2 tablespoons) at a time, until pureed consistency is achieved.
7. Using approximately 10 second intervals, process as long as necessary to eliminate all lumps:
    a. Stop the processor and scrape sides after each interval of processing.
    b. Typically, 1–2 rounds of processing and scraping will be needed.
    c. If you cannot process to smooth, remove obvious lumps with a spoon.
8. Evaluate to ensure compliance with IDDSI ④ Pureed requirements:
    a. No lumps and no separated water-thin liquids.
    b. Food sits on a mound above a dinner fork but does not drip or flow continuously through the fork.
    c. Easily separates and comes through the tines of a fork.
    d. Holds shape on a spoon, and slides off a teaspoon with little left—not sticky.
9. Remove from bowl and serve immediately, or separate into portions for storage in refrigerator or freezer.

Bonus presentation tip: Put ④ Pureed Peaches into a pastry bag with tip, or zip-style plastic bag. Use pastry tip or cut off corner of bag to pipe onto plate for improved presentation.

Warning: Fresh peaches need to have the pit removed and should be peeled thoroughly as the skins will not process well.

Pears

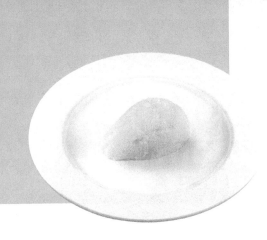

INGREDIENTS

- 16 oz. of pears—peeled and cored, rinsed and drained, as appropriate
- 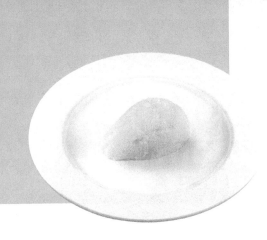 Extremely Thick Stock— see recipe on page 55

NOTES

The total amount of Extremely Thick Stock needed will vary on whether you start with canned or fresh pears. Canned pears will carry more liquid with them into the food processor than the fresh pears. Fresh pears should ripe and soft. On occasion, you may find that no additional Extremely Thick Stock is required to process properly. Rely on the process and your test results to ensure proper preparation.

DIRECTIONS

1. Add pears to food processor with sharp blade.
2. Put cover on processor.
3. Run processor for 15 seconds.
4. Open processor and inspect the contents of the processor bowl:
   a. Scrape sides and bottom of processor bowl.
   b. Remove any obviously tough or stringy pieces.
   c. If thin liquid begins to pool, drain or spoon out of processor.
5. Put cover on processor.
6. Start processor and add Extremely Thick Stock to the processor about 1 oz. (approximately 2 tablespoons) at a time, until pureed consistency is achieved.
7. Using approximately 10 second intervals, process as long as necessary to eliminate all lumps:
   a. Stop the processor and scrape sides after each interval of processing.
   b. Typically, 1–2 rounds of processing and scraping will be needed.
   c. If you cannot process to smooth, remove obvious lumps with a spoon.
8. Evaluate to ensure compliance with IDDSI Pureed requirements:
   a. No lumps and no separated water-thin liquids.
   b. Food sits on a mound above a dinner fork but does not drip or flow continuously through the fork.
   c. Easily separates and comes through the tines of a fork.
   d. Holds shape on a spoon, and slides off a teaspoon with little left—not sticky.
9. Remove from bowl and serve immediately, or separate into portions for storage in refrigerator or freezer.

Bonus presentation tip: Put Pureed Pears into a pastry bag with tip, or zip-style plastic bag. Use pastry tip or cut off corner of bag to pipe onto plate for improved presentation.

Warning: Fresh pears should have core, seeds and any tough parts removed and should be peeled thoroughly as the skins will not process well.

Buttered Noodles

INGREDIENTS

- 4 oz. (approx. 1 cup) dry pasta (elbow macaroni or angel hair/thin spaghetti are recommended)
- Water for boiling noodles — at least twice the amount recommended on the box
- 2 cups or more water for water bath
- Ice (optional)
- 4 oz. milk
- 2 tablespoons butter

NOTES

Our goal is to provide recipes that meet the IDDSI standards for at least 30 minutes after serving. The inherent starchiness of pasta made this a challenge to accomplish. In our quest for IDDSI-compliant pasta dishes, we tested pasta with a variety of cooking times—from al dente to falling apart. The process we settled upon is a bit different from traditional pasta instructions, but it does reliably remove as much of the sticky starch as possible. We boil the pasta for 30 minutes in an excess of water and rinse it to remove the released starch. Then we chill it in a water bath to stop the cooking process and keep the noodles moist and soft. After cooling, the pasta is ready to be processed and re-heated.

DIRECTIONS

1. Bring at least twice the package's recommended amount of water to a boil. The goal is to be sure every noodle is able to be fully cooked.
2. Add pasta and return to boil.
3. Stir occasionally.
4. Continue to boil for 30 minutes.
5. Drain pasta in colander.
6. Rinse pasta thoroughly with cold water in colander.
7. Chill pasta with water to refrigerator temperature—at or below 40°F (depending on which technique you use, this will take at least 30 minutes to 8 or more hours):
   a. If you are preparing pasta for more immediate use:
      i. Add ice and at least 4 cups of water to a large mixing bowl.
      ii. Add hot, drained, and rinsed pasta to ice water and mixing bowl.
      iii. Ensure the water level covers the pasta to chill and keep moist.
      iv. If hot pasta melts all the ice, add more ice to the bowl.
      v. Let pasta cool for at least 30 minutes.
   b. If you are preparing pasta for future use (within 2 days):
      i. Add hot, drained and rinsed pasta to an air tight container or zip-style plastic bag.
      ii. Add enough water to ensure the pasta is covered in water. The amount will vary based on your container size and shape, but it will likely be 2 or more cups of water.
      iii. Put in refrigerator for at least 8 hours.
      iv. Use within 2 days.
8. When ready to serve, drain cooled pasta in colander.
9. Add pasta, milk and butter to food processor with a sharp blade.
10. Put cover on processor and run for 20 seconds.
11. Remove cover. Scrape down sides. Remove any obviously stiff or undercooked pieces.
12. Put cover on processor and run for at least 60 seconds more, stopping occasionally to scrape down sides as needed.

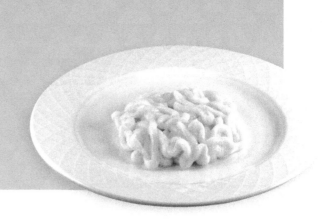

13. Evaluate to ensure compliance with IDDSI 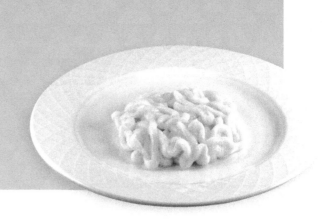 Pureed requirements:
    a. No lumps and no separated water-thin liquids.
    b. Food sits on a mound above a dinner fork but does not drip or flow continuously through the fork.
    c. Easily separates and comes through the tines of a fork.
    d. Holds shape on a spoon, and slides off a teaspoon with little left—not sticky.
14. If pasta is too sticky, add more milk, put cover on processor and run for a few seconds. Return to Step 12.
15. Move ④ Pureed pasta into pastry or freezer zip-style bag(s) with a plain pastry tip attached to store.
16. Refrigerate until ready to serve.
17. When serving, add noodles to a pastry bag with a round tip in place. Or simply add to a plastic bag and snip one corner off the bag. Pipe onto serving dish to give the appearance of noodles.
18. Use microwave or steamer (basket) to bring to serving temperature.

Homemade Shells & Cheese

INGREDIENTS

- 4 oz. dry shell pasta
- 4 oz. Velveeta® Original pasteurized recipe cheese product
- Water for boiling noodles — at least twice the amount recommended on the box
- 2 cups or more water for water bath
- Ice (optional)
- 2 oz. milk

NOTES

Our goal is to provide recipes that meet the IDDSI standards for at least 30 minutes after serving. The inherent starchiness of pasta made this a challenge to accomplish. In our quest for IDDSI-compliant pasta dishes, we tested pasta with a variety of cooking times—from al dente to falling apart. The process we settled upon is a bit different from traditional pasta instructions, but it does reliably remove as much of the sticky starch as possible. We boil the pasta for 30 minutes in an excess of water and rinse it to remove the released starch. Then we chill it in water to stop the cooking process and keep the noodles moist and soft. After cooling, the pasta is ready to be processed and re-heated.

DIRECTIONS

1. Bring at least twice the package's recommended amount of water to a boil. The goal is to be sure every noodle is able to be fully cooked.
2. Add pasta and return to boil.
3. Stir occasionally.
4. Continue to boil for 30 minutes.
5. Drain pasta in colander.
6. Rinse pasta thoroughly with cold water in colander.
7. Chill pasta with water to refrigerator temperature—at or below 40°F (depending on which technique you use, this will take at least 30 minutes to 8 or more hours):
   a. If you are preparing pasta for more immediate use:
      i. Add ice and at least 4 cups of water to a large mixing bowl.
      ii. Add hot, drained, and rinsed pasta to ice water and mixing bowl.
      iii. Ensure the water level covers the pasta to chill and keep moist.
      iv. If hot pasta melts all the ice, add more ice to the bowl.
      v. Let pasta cool for at least 30 minutes.
   b. If you are preparing pasta for future use (within 2 days):
      i. Add hot, drained and rinsed pasta to an air tight container or zip-style plastic bag.
      ii. Add enough water to ensure the pasta is covered in water. The amount will vary based on your container size and shape, but it will likely be 2 or more cups of water.
      iii. Put in refrigerator for at least 8 hours.
      iv. Use within 2 days.
8. When ready to serve, drain cooled pasta in colander.
9. Add pasta, milk and Velveeta® Original cheese product to food processor with a sharp blade.
10. Put cover on processor and run for 20 seconds.
11. Remove cover. Scrape down sides. Remove any obviously stiff or undercooked pieces.
12. Put cover on processor and run for at least 60 seconds, stopping occasionally to scrape down sides as needed.

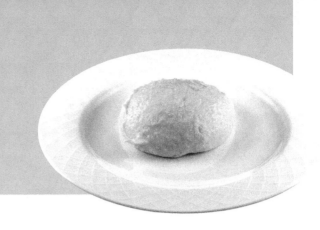

13. Evaluate to ensure compliance with IDDSI 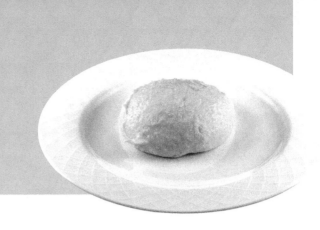 Pureed requirements:
    a. No lumps and no separated water-thin liquids.
    b. Food sits on a mound above a dinner fork but does not drip or flow continuously through the fork.
    c. Easily separates and comes through the tines of a fork.
    d. Holds shape on a spoon, and slides off a teaspoon with little left—not sticky.
14. If pasta is too sticky, add more milk, put cover on processor and run for a few seconds. Return to Step 12.
15. Move ④ Pureed pasta into pastry or freezer zip-style bag(s) with a plain pastry tip attached to store. (Pro tip: Using a shell pastry tip and technique can improve the appearance.)
16. Refrigerate until ready to serve.
17. To serve:
    a. Dispense ④ Pureed shells and cheese from bags in a shape you are comfortable with. Use shell tip to present shells. Or use a plain tip or a small corner cut from the bag to produce a spaghetti noodle shape and look.
    b. Use microwave or steamer to bring pasta up to serving temperature.

Velveeta® Shells & Cheese Original

INGREDIENTS

- 1 box Velveeta® Shells & Cheese—Original (12 oz.) (Each box contains shells and 1 liquid gold cheese sauce pouch)
- Water for boiling noodles — at least twice the amount recommended on the box
- 2 cups or more water for water bath
- Ice (optional)
- 2 oz. milk

NOTES

The "Liquid Gold" cheese sauce supplied in the box is very helpful in processing this dish because it is a ⚠ Extremely Thick liquid at room temperature.

Read "Notes" on the following page before proceeding.

DIRECTIONS

1. Bring water to a boil in a large pot.
2. Add pasta and return to boil.
3. Stir occasionally.
4. Continue to boil for 30 minutes.
5. Drain pasta in colander.
6. Rinse pasta thoroughly with cold water in colander.
7. Chill pasta with water to refrigerator temperature—at or below 40°F (depending on which technique you use, this will take at least 30 minutes to 8 or more hours):
   a. If you are preparing pasta for more immediate use:
      i. Add ice and at least 4 cups of water to a large mixing bowl.
      ii. Add hot, drained, and rinsed pasta to ice water and mixing bowl.
      iii. Ensure the water level covers the pasta to chill and keep moist.
      iv. If hot pasta melts all the ice, add more ice to the bowl.
      v. Let pasta cool for at least 30 minutes.
   b. If you are preparing pasta for future use (within 2 days):
      i. Add hot, drained and rinsed pasta to an air tight container or zip-style plastic bag.
      ii. Add enough water to ensure the pasta is covered in water. The amount will vary based on your container size and shape, but it will likely be 2 or more cups of water.
      iii. Put in refrigerator for at least 8 hours.
      iv. Use within 2 days.
8. When ready to serve, drain cooled pasta in colander.
9. Add pasta, milk and Liquid Gold cheese sauce pouch to food processor with a sharp blade.
10. Put cover on processor and run for 20 seconds.
11. Remove cover. Scrape down sides. Remove any obviously stiff or undercooked pieces.
12. Put cover on processor and run for at least 60 seconds, stopping occasionally to scrape down sides as needed.

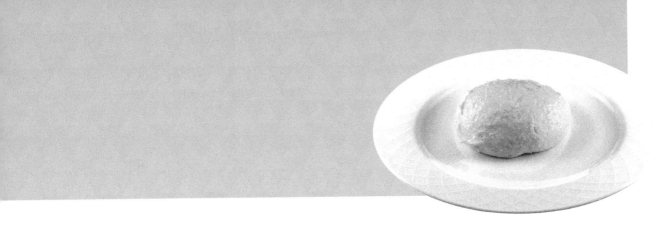

13. Evaluate to ensure compliance with IDDSI 4 Pureed requirements:
    a. No lumps and no separated water-thin liquids.
    b. Food sits on a mound above a dinner fork but does not drip or flow continuously through the fork.
    c. Easily separates and comes through the tines of a fork.
    d. Holds shape on a spoon, and slides off a teaspoon with little left—not sticky.
14. If pasta is too sticky, add more milk, put cover on processor and run for a few seconds. Return to Step 12.
15. Move 4 Pureed pasta into pastry or freezer zip-style bag(s) with a plain pastry tip attached to store. (Pro tip: Using a shell pastry tip and technique can improve the appearance.)
16. Refrigerate until ready to serve.
17. To serve:
    a. Dispense 4 Pureed shells and cheese from bags in a shape you are comfortable with. Use shell tip to present shells. Or a plain tip or a small corner cut to produce a spaghetti noodle shape and look.
    b. Use microwave or steamer to bring pasta up to serving temperature.

NOTES

Our goal is to provide recipes that meet the IDDSI standards for at least 30 minutes after serving. The inherent starchiness of pasta made this a challenge to accomplish. In our quest for IDDSI-compliant pasta dishes, we tested pasta with a variety of cooking times—from al dente to falling apart. The process we settled upon is a bit different from traditional pasta instructions, but it does reliably remove as much of the sticky starch as possible. We boil the pasta for 30 minutes in an excess of water and rinse it to remove the released starch. Then we chill it in water to stop the cooking process and keep the noodles moist and soft. After cooling, the pasta is ready to be processed and re-heated.

Spaghetti & Meatballs

INGREDIENTS

- 4 oz. (approx. 1 cup) dry pasta (elbow macaroni or angel hair/thin spaghetti are recommended)
- Water for boiling noodles — at least twice the amount recommended on the box
- 2 cups or more water for water bath
- Ice (optional)
- 4 oz. milk
- 16 oz. ⚠ Extremely Thick Marinara Sauce—see recipe on page 54
- 12–16 oz. ▼ Minced & Moist Meatballs—see recipe on page 124 (optional).

NOTES

This recipe is a capstone in our learning to process our favorite foods into IDDSI compliant dishes. We combine the processing of up to 3 separate components to produce a wonderful, tasty meal. Because of the time required to process the pasta, you will have time to make the sauce and the optional meatballs while the noodles are cooking and cooling.

Read "Notes" on the following page before proceeding.

DIRECTIONS

1. Bring at least twice the package's recommended amount of water to a boil. We want to be sure every noodle is able to be fully cooked.
2. Add pasta and return to boil.
3. Stir occasionally.
4. Continue to boil for 30 minutes.

While pasta is cooking, prepare ⚠ Extremely Thick Marinara Sauce and (optional ⚠ Pureed Meatballs.)

5. Drain pasta in colander.
6. Rinse pasta thoroughly with cold water in colander.
7. Chill pasta with water to refrigerator temperature—at or below 40°F (depending on which technique you use, this will take at least 30 minutes to 8 or more hours):
   a. If you are preparing pasta for more immediate use:
      i. Add ice and at least 4 cups of water to a large mixing bowl.
      ii. Add hot, drained, and rinsed pasta to ice water and mixing bowl.
      iii. Ensure the water level covers the pasta to chill and keep moist.
      iv. If hot pasta melts all the ice, add more ice to the bowl.
      v. Let pasta cool for at least 30 minutes.
   b. If you are preparing pasta for future use (within 2 days):
      i. Add hot, drained and rinsed pasta to an air tight container or zip-style plastic bag.
      ii. Add enough water to ensure the pasta is covered in water. The amount will vary based on your container size and shape, but it will likely be 2 or more cups of water.
      iii. Put in refrigerator for at least 8 hours.
      iv. Use within 2 days.
8. When ready to serve, drain cooled pasta in colander.
9. At this point, your next step depends on how you would like to serve the dish: the marinara sauce can be mixed with the noodles, or it can be served on top of them:
   a. For sauce premixed with the noodles, add pasta, 2 oz. of milk and 2 oz. of ⚠ Extremely Thick Marinara Sauce to processor with a sharp blade.
   b. For sauce on top presentation, add pasta and 4 oz. of milk to processor with a sharp blade.
10. Put cover on processor and run for 20 seconds.

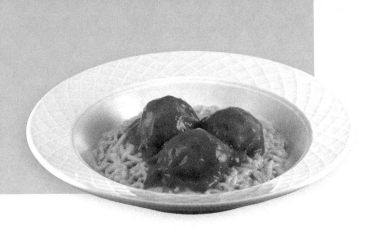

11. Remove cover. Scrape down sides. Remove any obviously stiff or undercooked pieces.
12. Put cover on processor and run for at least 60 seconds, stopping occasionally to scrape down sides as needed.
13. Evaluate to ensure compliance with IDDSI 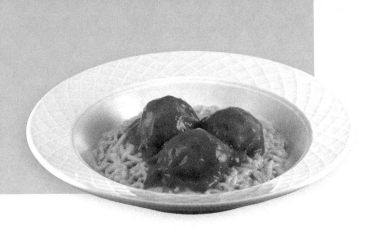 Pureed requirements:
    a. No lumps and no separated water-thin liquids.
    b. Food sits on a mound above a dinner fork but does not drip or flow continuously through the fork.
    c. Easily separates and comes through the tines of a fork.
    d. Holds shape on a spoon, and slides off a teaspoon with little left—not sticky.
14. If pasta is too sticky, add more ⃤ Extremely Thick Marinara Sauce OR milk, as appropriate to your noodle choice. Put cover on processor and run for a few seconds. Return to Step 12.
15. Move ▽ Pureed pasta into pastry or freezer zip-style bag(s) with a plain pastry tip attached to store.
16. Refrigerate until ready to serve.
17. To serve:
    a. Dispense ▽ Pureed pasta from bags to form long spaghetti noodle shapes:
        i. If using a disposable pastry or zip-style plastic bag(s), cut a small hole in one corner.
        ii. Squeeze bag(s) and move evenly back and forth about 3 or 4 inches above serving dish to make the spaghetti noodle shape.
    b. Layer on ⃤ Extremely Thick Marinara Sauce and ▽ Pureed Meatballs, as desired.
    c. Use microwave or steamer to bring pasta up to serving temperature.

NOTES

Our goal is to provide recipes that meet the IDDSI standards for at least 30 minutes after serving. The inherent starchiness of pasta made this a challenge to accomplish. In our quest for IDDSI-compliant pasta dishes, we tested pasta with a variety of cooking times—from al dente to falling apart. The process we settled upon is a bit different from traditional pasta instructions, but it does reliably remove as much of the sticky starch as possible. We boil the pasta for 30 minutes in an excess of water and rinse it to remove the released starch. Then we chill it in water to stop the cooking process and keep the noodles moist and soft. After cooling, the pasta is ready to be processed and re-heated.

Chocolate Raspberry Parfait

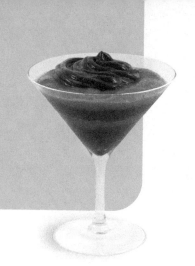

INGREDIENTS

- 1 cup raspberry gelatin, prepared according to package instructions
- 1 teaspoon whipped cream
- 1 cup chocolate pudding, prepared according to package instructions
- 24g SimplyThick® EasyMix™—this is can be achieved with:
  - 4 strokes from a pump bottle or;
  - 6 ▲ Slightly Thick packets (4g) or;
  - 4 ▲ Mildly Thick packets (6g) or;
  - 2 ▲ Moderately Thick packets (12g)

NOTES

Gelatin is a tricky food for dysphagia diets because it can melt into a thin liquid. And thickening the liquid before the gelatin sets won't work either.

We have found that processing gelatin with SimplyThick® EasyMix™ avoids both issues. The thickener thickens any loose liquids as it melts. Layering this with some pudding (which requires no additional processing) makes a fantastic dessert.

DIRECTIONS

1. Add raspberry gelatin, whipped cream and SimplyThick® EasyMix™ to food processor with sharp blade.
2. Put cover on processor.
3. Run processor for 15 seconds.
4. Open processor and inspect the contents of the processor bowl. Scrape sides and bottom of processor bowl.
5. If necessary, put cover on processor, run for an additional 10 seconds and return to Step 4.
6. Evaluate to ensure compliance with IDDSI ▽ Pureed requirements:
   a. No lumps and no separated water-thin liquids.
   b. Food sits on a mound above a dinner fork but does not drip or flow continuously through the fork.
   c. Easily separates and comes through the tines of a fork.
   d. Holds shape on a spoon, and slides off a teaspoon with little left—not sticky.
7. Fill serving dishes with alternating layers of processed gelatin and pudding.
8. Remove from bowl and serve immediately, or separate into portions for storage in refrigerator.

Bonus presentation tip: This looks great in fun, clear glassware!

Lemon Parfait

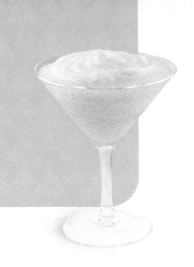

INGREDIENTS

- 1 cup lemon gelatin, prepared according to package instructions
- 1 cup lemon pudding, prepared according to package instructions
- 24g SimplyThick® EasyMix™— this is can be achieved with:
  - 4 strokes from a pump bottle or;
  - 6 ⚠ Slightly Thick packets (4g) or;
  - 4 ⚠ Mildly Thick packets (6g) or;
  - 2 ⚠ Moderately Thick packets (12g)

NOTES

Gelatin is a tricky food for dysphagia diets because it can melt into a thin liquid. And thickening the liquid before the gelatin sets won't work either.

We have found that processing gelatin with SimplyThick® EasyMix™ avoids both issues. The thickener thickens any loose liquids as it melts. Layering this with some pudding (which requires no additional processing) makes a fantastic dessert.

DIRECTIONS

1. Add lemon gelatin and SimplyThick® EasyMix™ to food processor with sharp blade.
2. Put cover on processor.
3. Run processor for 15 seconds.
4. Open processor and inspect the contents of the processor bowl. Scrape sides and bottom of processor bowl.
5. If necessary, put cover on processor, run for an additional 10 seconds and return to Step 4.
6. Evaluate to ensure compliance with IDDSI ▽4 Pureed requirements:
   a. No lumps and no separated water-thin liquids.
   b. Food sits on a mound above a dinner fork but does not drip or flow continuously through the fork.
   c. Easily separates and comes through the tines of a fork.
   d. Holds shape on a spoon, and slides off a teaspoon with little left—not sticky.
7. Fill serving dishes with alternating layers of processed gelatin and pudding.
8. Remove from bowl and serve immediately, or separate into portions for storage in refrigerator.

Bonus presentation tip: This looks great in fun, clear glassware!

MINCED & MOIST

LEVEL 5 – MINCED & MOIST

Description/characteristics

- Can be eaten with a fork or spoon
- Can be eaten with chopsticks in some cases, if the individual has very good hand control
- Can be scooped and shaped (e.g. into a ball shape) on a plate
- Soft and moist with no separated thin liquid
- Small lumps visible within the food
  - Pediatric: equal to or less than 2 mm wide and no longer than 8 mm in length
  - Adult: equal to or less than 4 mm wide and no longer than 15 mm in length
- Lumps are easy to squash with tongue

Physiological rationale for this level of thickness

- Biting is not required
- Minimal chewing is required
- Tongue force alone can be used to separate the soft small particles in this texture
- Tongue force is required to move the bolus
- Pain or fatigue when chewing
- Missing teeth, poorly fitting dentures

Although descriptions are provided, use IDDSI Testing methods to decide if the food meets IDDSI ▽5 Minced & Moist guidelines for adults.

NOTES AND TIPS ON ▽5 MINCED & MOIST

Not all foods in the ▽4 Pureed section will be found here. Some foods, like fruit, have so much fluid inside that they naturally pass the ▽5 Minced & Moist stage and go directly to ▽4 Pureed in a food processor. It may be possible to achieve ▽5 Minced & Moist with these items with a knife, but this technique seems outside the scope and spirit of our recipes.

If you or your loved one can eat ▽5 Minced & Moist, they can also eat any of the ▽4 Pureed foods. So you can incorporate any of the ▽4 Pureed recipes into a ▽5 Minced & Moist diet.

THE RECIPES

Beef (Steak or Roast)

Ground Beef

Shredded Beef

Meatloaf

Meatballs

Ham

Pulled Pork

Pork Chops or Pork Loin

Chicken

Turkey

Breaded Fish or Fish Sticks

Sauteed Fish

Scrambled Eggs

Egg Salad

Potato Salad

Chicken Salad

Tuna Salad

Coleslaw

Carrots

Cauliflower

Broccoli

Butternut Squash

Green Beans

Peas

Snow or Sugarsnap Peas

Spinach

Buttered Noodles

Homemade Shells & Cheese

Velveeta® Shells & Cheese Original

Spaghetti & Meatballs

Beef (Steak or Roast)

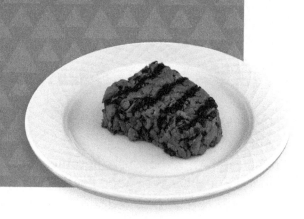

INGREDIENTS

- 16 oz. cooked and drained beef (hot or cold meat can be used—skin, bones, cartilage, gristle, excessive fat and crusty edges must be removed)
- ⚠ Extremely Thick Stock— see recipe on page 55

NOTES

Each batch of meat will behave a little differently and this recipe is designed to be flexible and allow you to ensure compliance with IDDSI guidelines.

This process will work with both hot and cold cooked beef. When working with hot foods that contain fat/oil, you will likely need less ⚠ Extremely Thick Stock because the hot fat/oil will help lubricate the meat and achieve ▼ Minced & Moist results. When working with cold meat, the fat behaves more like a solid and typically requires a little more liquid to achieve the desired ▼ Minced & Moist results.

About half of the time, you will NOT need to add any ⚠ Extremely Thick Stock to the meat. Rely on the process and your test results to ensure proper preparation.

DIRECTIONS

1. Add cooked beef into a food processor with sharp blade.
2. Put cover on processor.
3. Run processor for 10 seconds.
4. Open processor and evaluate meat for compliance with the size requirements for IDDSI ▼ Minced & Moist:
   a. Remove any obviously undercooked, tough or stringy pieces.
   b. If all pieces are equal to or smaller than 4 mm x 4 mm x 15 mm, go to Step 5.
   c. If not, scrape all meat off the side of the processor bowl and return to Step 2.
5. Put processed meat into a mixing bowl and stir with a spatula. Evaluate the moisture level and whether water-thin liquids are weeping or separating from the beef:
   a. If water-thin liquid is visible in the bottom of the bowl or is separating from the meat, go to Step 6.
   b. If water-thin liquid is not visible and the meat appears dry and will not stick together, go to Step 6.
   c. If water-thin liquid is not present and the meat is moist and holds together, go to Step 7.
6. If water-thin liquid is present or the meat is too dry, it is necessary to add some ⚠ Extremely Thick Stock to the meat to comply with IDDSI standards:
   a. If present, remove excess water-thin liquid with a spoon.
   b. Add small amounts of ⚠ Extremely Thick Stock to the meat and stir with spatula to thoroughly combine liquids and solids.
   c. Continue adding small amounts of ⚠ Extremely Thick Stock until meat is moist and no water-thin liquid is separating.
7. Evaluate to ensure compliance with IDDSI ▼ Minced & Moist requirements:
   a. No separated water-thin liquids.
   b. Easily mashed with little pressure from a fork.
   c. Easily separates and comes through the tines of a fork.
   d. Holds its shape and slides off with little food left on a teaspoon.
8. Remove from bowl and serve, or separate into portions for storage.

Ground Beef

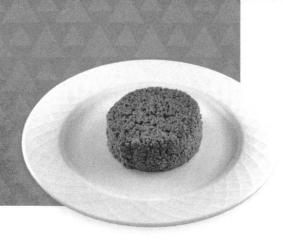

INGREDIENTS

- 16 oz. cooked ground beef, drained of grease (hot or cold meat can be used—bones and gristle must be removed)
- 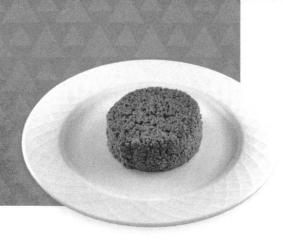 Extremely Thick Stock—see recipe on page 55

NOTES

You can follow this process with ground meat substitutes as well.

Each batch of meat will behave a little differently and this recipe is designed to be flexible and allow you to ensure compliance with IDDSI guidelines.

This process will work with both hot and cold ground beef. When working with hot foods that contain fat/oil, you will likely need less ⚠ Extremely Thick Stock because the hot fat/oil will help lubricate the meat and achieve ▼ Minced & Moist results. When working with cold meat, the fat behaves more like a solid and typically requires a little more liquid to achieve the desired ▼ Minced & Moist results.

About half of the time, you will NOT need to add any ⚠ Extremely Thick Stock to the meat. Rely on the process and your test results to ensure proper preparation.

DIRECTIONS

1. Put ground beef into food processor with sharp blade.
2. Put cover on processor.
3. Run processor for 15 seconds.
4. Open processor and evaluate ground beef for compliance with the size requirements for IDDSI ▼ Minced & Moist:
   a. Remove any obviously undercooked, tough or stringy pieces.
   b. If all pieces are equal to or smaller than 4 mm x 4 mm x 15 mm, go to step 5.
   c. If not, scrape all meat off the side of the processor bowl and return to Step 2.
5. Put processed meat into a mixing bowl and stir with a spatula. Evaluate the moisture level and whether water-thin liquids are weeping or separating from the beef:
   a. If water-thin liquid is visible in the bottom of the bowl or is separating from the ground beef, go to step 6.
   b. If water-thin liquid is not visible and the ground beef appears dry and will not hold together, go to step 6.
   c. If water-thin liquid is not present and the ground beef is moist and holds together, go to step 7. With ground beef this will rarely, if ever be the case.
6. If water-thin liquid is present or the meat is too dry, it is necessary to add some ⚠ Extremely Thick Stock to the meat to comply with IDDSI standards:
   a. If present, remove excess water-thin liquid with a spoon.
   b. Add small amounts of ⚠ Extremely Thick Stock to the meat and stir with spatula to thoroughly combine liquids and solids.
   c. Continue adding small amounts of ⚠ Extremely Thick Stock until meat is moist and no water-thin liquid is separating.
7. Evaluate to ensure compliance with IDDSI ▼ Minced & Moist requirements:
   a. No separated water-thin liquids.
   b. Easily mashed with little pressure from a fork.
   c. Easily separates and comes through the tines of a fork.
   d. Holds its shape and slides off with little food left on a teaspoon.
8. Remove from bowl and serve, or separate into portions for storage.

Shredded Beef

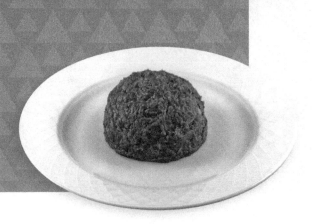

INGREDIENTS

- 16 oz. cooked shredded beef, drained of excess drippings (hot or cold meat can be used—skin, bones and cartilage must be removed)
- ⒋ Extremely Thick Stock— see recipe on page 55

NOTES

Each batch of meat will behave a little differently and this recipe is designed to be flexible and allow you to ensure compliance with IDDSI guidelines.

This process will work with both hot and cold shredded beef. When working with hot foods that contain fat/oil, you will likely need less ⒋ Extremely Thick Stock because the hot fat/oil will help lubricate the meat and achieve ⑤ Minced & Moist results. When working with cold meat, the fat behaves more like a solid and typically requires a little more liquid to achieve the desired ⑤ Minced & Moist results.

About half of the time, you will NOT need to add any ⒋ Extremely Thick Stock to the meat. Rely on the process and your test results to ensure proper preparation.

DIRECTIONS

1. Add shredded beef to food processor with sharp blade.
2. Put cover on processor.
3. Run processor for 10 seconds.
4. Open processor and evaluate meat for compliance with the size requirements for IDDSI ⑤ Minced & Moist:
   a. Remove any obviously undercooked, tough or stringy pieces.
   b. If all pieces are equal to or smaller than 4 mm x 4 mm x 15 mm, go to Step 5.
   c. If not, scrape all meat off the side of the processor bowl and return to Step 2.
5. Put processed meat into a mixing bowl and stir with a spatula. Evaluate the moisture level and whether water-thin liquids are weeping or separating from the beef:
   a. If water-thin liquid is visible in the bottom of the bowl or is separating from the meat, go to Step 6.
   b. If water-thin liquid is not visible and the meat appears dry and will not stick together, go to Step 6.
   c. If water-thin liquid is not present and the meat is moist and holds together, go to Step 7.
6. If water-thin liquid is present or the meat is too dry, it is necessary to add some ⒋ Extremely Thick Stock to the meat to comply with IDDSI standards:
   a. Remove excess water-thin liquid with a spoon.
   b. Add small amounts of ⒋ Extremely Thick Stock to the meat and stir with spatula to thoroughly combine liquids and solids.
   c. Continue adding small amounts of ⒋ Extremely Thick Stock until meat is moist and no water-thin liquid is separating.
7. Evaluate to ensure compliance with IDDSI ⑤ Minced & Moist requirements:
   a. No separated water-thin liquids.
   b. Easily mashed with little pressure from a fork.
   c. Easily separates and comes through the tines of a fork.
   d. Holds its shape and slides off with little food left on a teaspoon.
8. Remove from bowl and serve, or separate into portions for storage.

Meatloaf

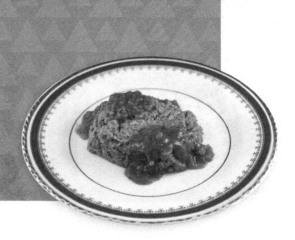

INGREDIENTS

- 13.2 oz. Stouffer's® meatloaf or equivalent—microwaved per instructions or fresh made from scratch meatloaf
- Depending on end use, 4 oz. 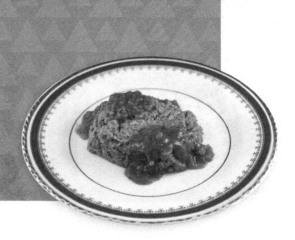 Extremely Thick Sauce or Stock— see Basic Sauce recipe on page 51 for ketchup glaze or BBQ sauce, or 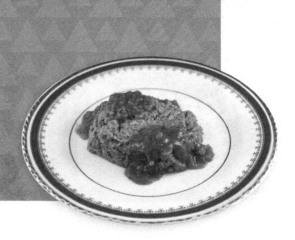 Extremely Thick Stock recipe on page 55

NOTES

Since it is commonly available nationwide, most of our testing used Stouffer's® brand frozen meatloaf. Similar results were obtained with other frozen meatloaf brands. Other meatloaf brands may behave a little differently, however this recipe is designed to be flexible and allow you to ensure compliance with IDDSI guidelines. If you make meatloaf from scratch, consider using a food processor as you make the meatloaf. With the added mechanical processing, fresh ingredients, and never having been frozen, we found fresh-made meatloaf from scratch was already in compliance with IDDSI 5 Minced & Moist requirements.

DIRECTIONS

1. Drain any thin sauce or drippings and add cooked meatloaf to food processor with sharp blade.
2. Put cover on processor.
3. Run processor for 10 seconds.
4. Open processor and evaluate meatloaf for compliance with the size requirements for IDDSI 5 Minced & Moist:
   a. Remove any obviously undercooked, tough or stringy pieces.
   b. If all pieces are equal to or smaller than 4 mm x 4 mm x 15 mm, go to Step 5.
   c. If not, scrape all meatloaf off the side of processor bowl and return to Step 2.
5. Put processed meatloaf into a mixing bowl and stir with a spatula. Evaluate the moisture level and whether water-thin liquids are weeping or separating from the meatloaf:
   a. If water-thin liquid is visible in the bottom of the bowl or is separating from the meatloaf, go to Step 6.
   b. If water-thin liquid is not visible and the meatloaf appears dry and will not stick together, go to Step 6.
   c. If water-thin liquid is not present and the meatloaf is moist and holds together, go to Step 7.
6. If water-thin liquid is present or the meatloaf is too dry, it is necessary to add some 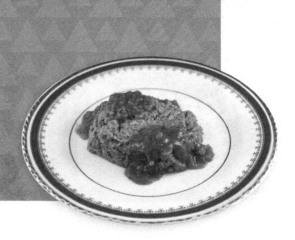 Extremely Thick Sauce or Stock to the meatloaf to comply with IDDSI standards:
   a. Remove excess water-thin liquid with a spoon.
   b. Add small amounts of 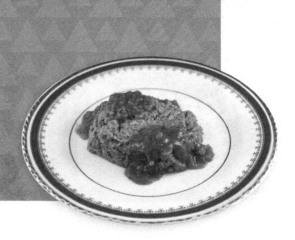 Extremely Thick Sauce or Stock (as preferred) to the meatloaf and stir with spatula to thoroughly combine liquids and solids.
   c. Continue adding small amounts of 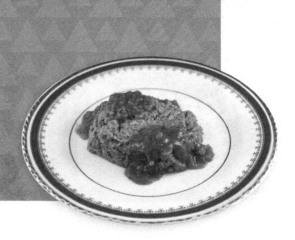 Extremely Thick Sauce or Stock until meatloaf is moist and no water-thin liquid is separating.
7. Evaluate to ensure compliance with IDDSI 5 Minced & Moist requirements:
   a. No separated water-thin liquids.
   b. Easily mashed with little pressure from a fork.
   c. Easily separates and comes through the tines of a fork.
   d. Holds its shape and slides off with little food left on a teaspoon.
8. Remove from bowl and serve, or separate into portions for storage.

Meatballs

INGREDIENTS

- 12–16 oz. frozen or fresh made from scratch meatballs — cooked per package instructions
- Depending on end use, 4 oz. △ Extremely Thick Sauce or Stock— see Marinara Sauce recipe on page 54, or △ Extremely Thick Stock recipe on page 55

NOTES

These meatballs offer a flexible base for a variety of dishes. They can be used as a component to a pasta dish, a topping for ▽ Pureed bread or simply covered with an appropriately thickened sauce. There are a variety of frozen meatballs available and each may behave a little differently, however this recipe is designed to be flexible and allow you to ensure compliance with IDDSI guidelines.

If you make meatballs from scratch, consider using a food processor as you make the meatballs. With the added mechanical processing, fresh ingredients, and never having been frozen, fresh-made meatballs from scratch may already be in compliance with IDDSI ▽ Minced & Moist requirements when you are finished making them.

DIRECTIONS

1. Drain any thin sauce or drippings and add cooked meatballs to food processor with sharp blade.
2. Put cover on processor.
3. Run processor for 10 seconds.
4. Open processor and evaluate meat for compliance with the size requirements for IDDSI ▽ Minced & Moist:
   a. Remove any obviously undercooked, tough or stringy pieces.
   b. If all pieces are equal to or smaller than 4 mm x 4 mm x 15 mm, go to Step 5.
   c. If not, scrape all meat off the side of the processor bowl and return to Step 2.
5. Put processed meatballs into a mixing bowl and stir with a spatula. Evaluate the moisture level and whether water-thin liquids are weeping or separating from the meatballs:
   a. If water-thin liquid is visible in the bottom of the bowl or is separating from the meat, go to Step 6.
   b. If water-thin liquid is not visible and the meat appears dry and will not stick together, go to Step 6.
   c. If water-thin liquid is not present and the meat is moist and holds together, go to Step 7.
6. If water-thin liquid is present or the meat is too dry, it is necessary to add some △ Extremely Thick Sauce or Stock to the meatballs to comply with IDDSI standards:
   a. Remove excess water-thin liquid with a spoon.
   b. Add small amounts of △ Extremely Thick Sauce or Stock (as preferred) to the meatballs and stir with spatula to thoroughly combine liquids and solids.
   c. Continue adding small amounts of △ Extremely Thick Sauce or Stock until meat is moist and no water-thin liquid is separating.
7. Evaluate to ensure compliance with IDDSI ▽ Minced & Moist requirements:
   a. No separated water-thin liquids.
   b. Easily mashed with little pressure from a fork.
   c. Easily separates and comes through the tines of a fork.
   d. Holds its shape and slides off with little food left on a teaspoon.
8. Remove from bowl and form 1½ inch meatball shapes with clean sanitary hands or gloved hands.
9. Add to final dish, or store in refrigerator for later use.

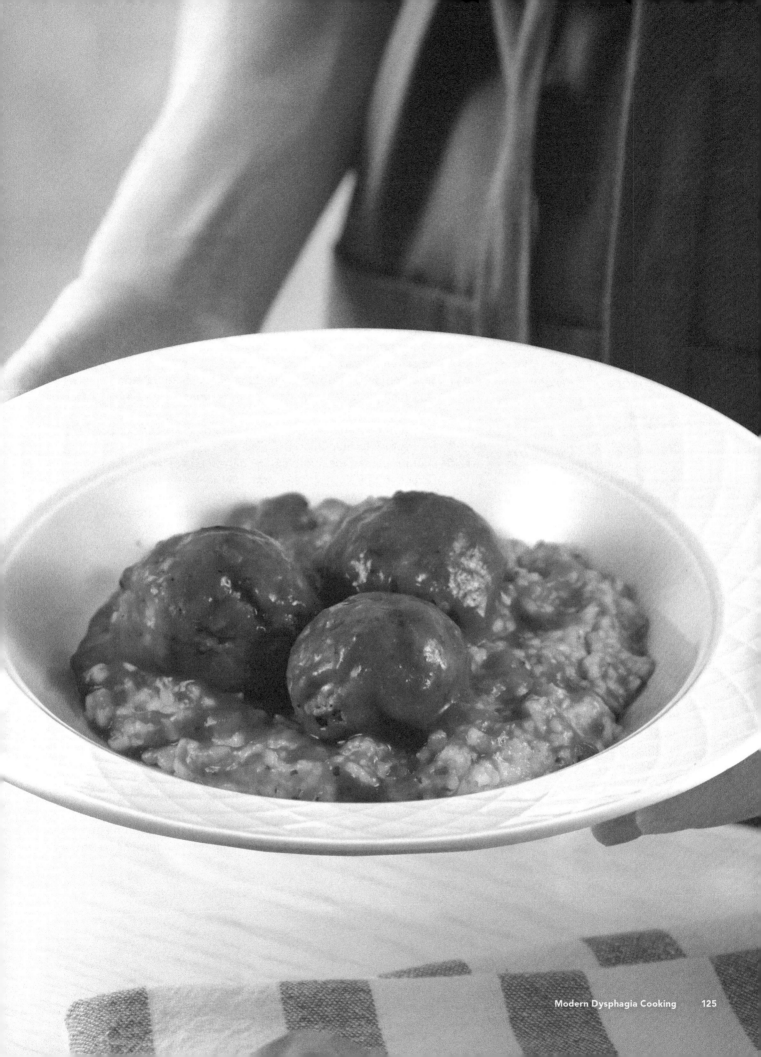

Ham

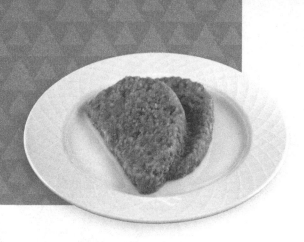

INGREDIENTS

- 16 oz. cooked ham, drained of excess drippings (hot or cold meat can be used—skin, bones and cartilage must be removed)
- 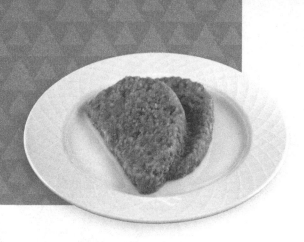 Extremely Thick Stock— see recipe on page 55

NOTES

We worked with convenience/ pre-packaged sliced or diced ham. Each batch of meat will behave a little differently and this recipe is designed to be flexible and allow you to ensure compliance with IDDSI guidelines. This process will work with both hot and cold cooked ham. When working with hot foods that contain fat/oil, you will likely need less Extremely Thick Stock because the hot fat/oil will help lubricate the meat and achieve Minced & Moist results. When working with cold meat, the fat/oil behaves more like a solid and typically requires a little more liquid to achieve the desired Minced & Moist results.

DIRECTIONS

1. Add ham to a food processor with sharp blade.
2. Put cover on processor.
3. Run processor for 10 seconds.
4. Open processor and evaluate meat for compliance with the size requirements for IDDSI 5 Minced & Moist:
   a. Remove any obviously undercooked, tough or stringy pieces.
   b. If all pieces are equal to or smaller than 4 mm x 4 mm x 15 mm, go to Step 5.
   c. If not, scrape all meat off the side of the processor bowl and return to Step 2.
5. Put processed meat into a mixing bowl and stir with a spatula. Evaluate the moisture level and whether water-thin liquids are weeping or separating from the ham:
   a. If water-thin liquid is visible in the bottom of the bowl or is separating from the meat, go to Step 6.
   b. If water-thin liquid is not visible and the meat appears dry and will not stick together, go to Step 6.
   c. If water-thin liquid is not present and the meat is moist and holds together, go to Step 7.
6. If water-thin liquid is present or the meat is too dry, it is necessary to add some Extremely Thick Stock to the meat to comply with IDDSI standards:
   a. If present, remove excess water-thin liquid with a spoon.
   b. Add small amounts of Extremely Thick Stock to the meat and stir with spatula to thoroughly combine liquids and solids.
   c. Continue adding small amounts of Extremely Thick Stock until meat is moist and no water-thin liquid is separating.
7. Evaluate to ensure compliance with IDDSI 5 Minced & Moist requirements:
   a. No separated water-thin liquids.
   b. Easily mashed with little pressure from a fork.
   c. Easily separates and comes through the tines of a fork.
   d. Holds its shape and slides off with little food left on a teaspoon.
8. Remove from bowl and serve, or separate into portions for storage.

Pulled Pork

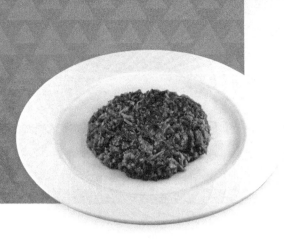

INGREDIENTS

- 16 oz. cooked pulled pork, drained of excess drippings (hot or cold meat can be used—skin, bones and cartilage must be removed)
- ④ Extremely Thick Stock—see recipe on page 55

NOTES

Each batch of meat will behave a little differently and this recipe is designed to be flexible and allow you to ensure compliance with IDDSI guidelines.

This process will work with both hot and cold pulled pork. When working with hot foods that contain fat/oil, you will likely need less ④ Extremely Thick Stock because the hot fat/oil will help lubricate the meat and achieve ⑤ Minced & Moist results. When working with cold meat, the fat behaves more like a solid and typically requires a little more liquid to achieve the desired ⑤ Minced & Moist results.

About half of the time, you will NOT need to add any ④ Extremely Thick Stock to the meat. Rely on the process and your test results to ensure proper preparation.

DIRECTIONS

1. Add pulled pork to a food processor with sharp blade.
2. Put cover on processor.
3. Run processor for 10 seconds.
4. Open processor and evaluate meat for compliance with the size requirements for IDDSI ⑤ Minced & Moist:
   a. Remove any obviously undercooked, tough or stringy pieces
   b. If all pieces are equal to or smaller than 4 mm x 4 mm x 15 mm, go to Step 5.
   c. If not, scrape all meat off the side of the processor bowl and return to Step 2.
5. Put processed meat into a mixing bowl and stir with a spatula. Evaluate the moisture level and whether water-thin liquids are weeping or separating from the pork:
   a. If water-thin liquid is visible in the bottom of the bowl or is separating from the meat, go to Step 6.
   b. If water-thin liquid is not visible and the meat appears dry and will not stick together, go to Step 6.
   c. If water-thin liquid is not present and the meat is moist and holds together, go to Step 7.
6. If water-thin liquid is present or the meat is too dry, it is necessary to add some ④ Extremely Thick Stock to the meat to comply with IDDSI standards:
   a. Remove excess water-thin liquid with a spoon.
   b. Add small amounts of ④ Extremely Thick Stock to the meat and stir with spatula to thoroughly combine liquids and solids.
   c. Continue adding small amounts of ④ Extremely Thick Stock until meat is moist and no water-thin liquid is separating.
7. Evaluate to ensure compliance with IDDSI ⑤ Minced & Moist requirements:
   a. No separated water-thin liquids.
   b. Easily mashed with little pressure from a fork.
   c. Easily separates and comes through the tines of a fork.
   d. Holds its shape and slides off with little food left on a teaspoon.
8. Remove from bowl and serve, or separate into portions for storage.

Pork Chops or Pork Loin

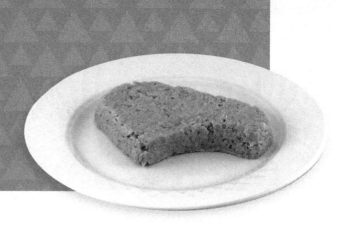

INGREDIENTS

- 16 oz. cooked pork chops or loin (hot or cold meat can be used—skin, bones and cartilage must be removed)
- 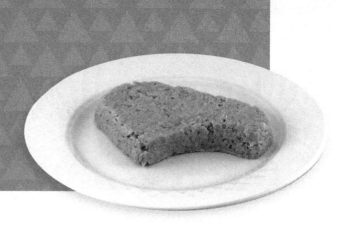 Extremely Thick Stock— see recipe on page 55

NOTES

Each batch of meat will behave a little differently and this recipe is designed to be flexible and allow you to ensure compliance with IDDSI guidelines.

This process will work with both hot and cold cooked pork chops or pork loin. When working with hot foods that contain fat/oil, you will likely need less ④ Extremely Thick Stock because the hot fat/oil will help lubricate the meat and achieve ⑤ Minced & Moist results. When working with cold meat the fat/oil behaves more like a solid and typically requires a little more liquid to achieve the desired ⑤ Minced & Moist results.

DIRECTIONS

1. Add cooked pork chops or pork loin to a food processor with sharp blade.
2. Put cover on processor.
3. Run processor for 10 seconds.
4. Open processor and evaluate meat for compliance with the size requirements for IDDSI ⑤ Minced & Moist:
   a. Remove any obviously undercooked, tough or stringy pieces.
   b. If all pieces are equal to or smaller than 4 mm x 4 mm x 15 mm, go to Step 5.
   c. If not, scrape all meat off the side of the processor bowl and return to Step 2.
5. Put processed meat into a mixing bowl and stir with a spatula. Evaluate the moisture level and whether water-thin liquids are weeping or separating from the pork:
   a. If water-thin liquid is visible in the bottom of the bowl or is separating from the meat, go to Step 6.
   b. If water-thin liquid is not visible and the meat appears dry and will not stick together, go to Step 6.
   c. If water-thin liquid is not present and the meat is moist and holds together, go to Step 7.
6. If thin liquid is present or the meat is too dry, it is necessary to add some ④ Extremely Thick Stock to the meat to comply with IDDSI standards:
   a. If present, remove excess thin liquid with a spoon.
   b. Add small amounts of ④ Extremely Thick Stock to the meat and stir with spatula to thoroughly combine liquids and solids.
   c. Continue adding small amounts of ④ Extremely Thick Stock until meat is moist and no thin liquid is separating.
7. Evaluate to ensure compliance with IDDSI ⑤ Minced & Moist requirements:
   a. No separated water-thin liquids.
   b. Easily mashed with little pressure from a fork.
   c. Easily separates and comes through the tines of a fork.
   d. Holds its shape and slides off with little food left on a teaspoon.
8. Remove from bowl and serve, or separate into portions for storage.

Chicken

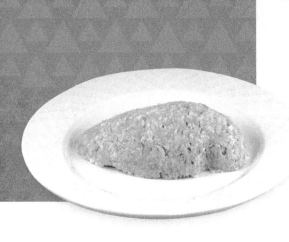

INGREDIENTS

- 16 oz. cooked and drained chicken (hot or cold meat can be used—skin, bones and cartilage must be removed)
- ▲ Extremely Thick Stock— see recipe on page 55

NOTES

Each batch of meat will behave a little differently and this recipe is designed to be flexible to ensure compliance with IDDSI guidelines.

This process will work with both hot and cold cooked chicken. When working with hot foods that contain fat/oil, you will likely need less ▲ Extremely Thick Stock because the hot fat/oil will help lubricate the meat and achieve ▼ Minced & Moist results. When working with cold meat, the fat behaves more like a solid and typically requires a little more liquid to achieve the desired ▼ Minced & Moist results.

DIRECTIONS

1. Add cooked chicken to a food processor with sharp blade.
2. Put cover on processor.
3. Run processor for 10 seconds.
4. Open processor and evaluate meat for compliance with the size requirements for IDDSI ▼ Minced & Moist:
   a. Remove any obviously undercooked, tough or stringy pieces.
   b. If all pieces are equal to or smaller than 4 mm x 4 mm x 15 mm, go to Step 5.
   c. If not, scrape all meat off the side of the processor bowl and return to Step 2.
5. Put processed meat into a mixing bowl and stir with a spatula. Evaluate the moisture level and whether water-thin liquids are weeping or separating from the chicken:
   a. If water-thin liquid is visible in the bottom of the bowl or is separating from the meat, go to Step 6.
   b. If water-thin liquid is not visible and the meat appears dry and will not stick together, go to Step 6.
   c. If water-thin liquid is not present and the meat is moist and holds together, go to Step 7.
6. If water-thin liquid is present or the meat is too dry, it is necessary to add some ▲ Extremely Thick Stock to the meat to comply with IDDSI standards:
   a. If present, remove excess water-thin liquid with a spoon.
   b. Add small amounts of ▲ Extremely Thick Stock to the meat and stir with spatula to thoroughly combine liquids and solids.
   c. Continue adding small amounts of ▲ Extremely Thick Stock until meat is moist and no water-thin liquid is separating.
7. Evaluate to ensure compliance with IDDSI ▼ Minced & Moist requirements:
   a. No separated water-thin liquids.
   b. Easily mashed with little pressure from a fork.
   c. Easily separates and comes through the tines of a fork.
   d. Holds its shape and slides off with little food left on a teaspoon.
8. Remove from bowl and serve, or separate into portions for storage.

Bonus presentation tip: Use a food form—see page 34.

Turkey

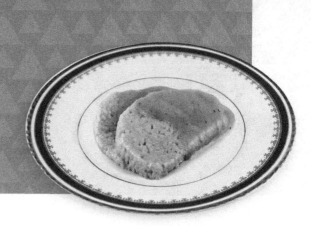

INGREDIENTS

- 16 oz. cooked turkey meat*, drained of excess drippings (hot or cold meat can be used—skin and bones must be removed)
- ⚠ Extremely Thick Stock— see recipe on page 55

NOTES

Each batch of meat will behave a little differently and this recipe is designed to be flexible to ensure compliance with IDDSI guidelines.

This process will work with both hot and cold cooked turkey. When working with hot foods that contain fat/oil, you will likely need less ⚠ Extremely Thick Stock because the hot fat/oil will help lubricate the meat and achieve 5 Minced & Moist results. When working with cold meat, the fat behaves more like a solid and typically requires a little more liquid to achieve the desired 5 Minced & Moist results.

On occasion, you will NOT need to add any ⚠ Extremely Thick Stock to the turkey. Rely on the process and your test results to ensure proper preparation.

DIRECTIONS

1. Add cooked turkey to a food processor with sharp blade.
2. Put cover on processor.
3. Run processor for 10 seconds.
4. Open processor and evaluate meat for compliance with the size requirements for IDDSI 5 Minced & Moist:
   a. Remove any obviously undercooked, tough or stringy pieces
   b. If all pieces are equal to or smaller than 4 mm x 4 mm x 15 mm, go to Step 5.
   c. If not, scrape all meat off the side of the processor bowl and return to Step 2.
5. Put processed meat into a mixing bowl and stir with a spatula. Evaluate the moisture level and whether water-thin liquids are weeping or separating from the turkey:
   a. If water-thin liquid is visible in the bottom of the bowl or is separating from the meat, go to Step 6.
   b. If water-thin liquid is not visible and the meat appears dry and will not stick together, go to Step 6.
   c. If water-thin liquid is not present and the meat is moist and holds together, go to Step 7.
6. If water-thin liquid is present or the meat is too dry, it is necessary to add some ⚠ Extremely Thick Stock to the meat to comply with IDDSI standards:
   a. If present, remove excess water-thin liquid with a spoon.
   b. Add small amounts of ⚠ Extremely Thick Stock to the meat and stir with spatula to thoroughly combine liquids and solids.
   c. Continue adding small amounts of ⚠ Extremely Thick Stock until meat is moist and no water-thin liquid is separating.
7. Evaluate to ensure compliance with IDDSI 5 Minced & Moist requirements:
   a. No separated water-thin liquids.
   b. Easily mashed with little pressure from a fork.
   c. Easily separates and comes through the tines of a fork.
   d. Holds its shape and slides off with little food left on a teaspoon.
8. Remove from bowl and serve, or separate into portions for storage.

*Cooked turkey meat includes sandwich meat and other packaged and cooked turkey meat.

MINCED & MOIST

Breaded Fish or Fish Sticks

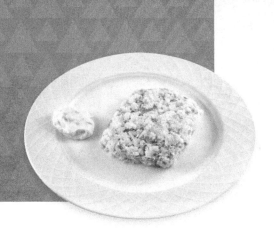

INGREDIENTS

- 16 oz. cooked frozen "beer battered" cod fillets, or breaded fish sticks or equivalent—cooked according to the manufacturer's instructions and still warm or hot
- ▲ Extremely Thick Stock— see recipe on page 55

NOTES

We DO NOT RECOMMEND storing portions of ▼ Minced & Moist breaded fish for later use. Our testers attempted to reheat portions of processed breaded fish that were stored in the refrigerator and freezer. The reheated stored portions were NOT able to pass IDDSI tests when reheated. The breading component became too sticky.

DIRECTIONS

1. Within 15 minutes of finishing cooking, put hot breaded fish into food processor with sharp blade. (Note: If breaded fish sits too long before processing, the breading will get gummy.)
2. Put cover on processor.
3. Run processor for 15 seconds.
4. Open processor and evaluate hot breaded fish for compliance with the size requirements for IDDSI ▼ Minced & Moist:
   a. Remove any obviously burnt, extra crispy, undercooked, tough or stringy pieces.
   b. If all pieces are equal to or smaller than 4 mm x 4 mm x 15 mm, go to step 5.
   c. If not, scrape all meat and batter off the side of processor bowl and return to Step 2.
5. Put processed hot breaded fish into a mixing bowl and stir with a spatula. Evaluate the moisture level, presence of water-thin liquid and cohesiveness:
   a. If water-thin liquid is visible in the bottom of the bowl or is separating from the hot breaded fish, go to step 6.
   b. If water-thin liquid is not visible and the hot breaded fish appears dry and will not hold together, go to step 6.
   c. If water-thin liquid is not present and the hot breaded fish is moist and holds together, go to step 7.
6. If water-thin liquid is present or the hot breaded fish is too dry, it is necessary to add some ▲ Thickened Stock to comply with IDDSI standards:
   a. Remove any excess water-thin liquid with a spoon.
   b. Add small amounts of ▲ Thickened Stock to the hot breaded fish and stir with spatula to thoroughly combine liquids and solids.
   c. Continue adding small amounts until hot breaded fish is moist and no water-thin liquid is separating.
7. Evaluate to ensure compliance with IDDSI ▼ Minced & Moist requirements:
   a. No separated water-thin liquids.
   b. Easily mashed with little pressure from a fork.
   c. Easily separates and comes through the tines of a fork.
   d. Holds its shape and slides off with little food left on a teaspoon.
8. Remove from bowl and serve immediately. Do NOT store for later use.

Sauteed Fish

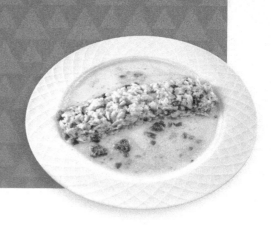

INGREDIENTS

- 16 oz. fish fillets, sauteed and "fork tender," drained of water-thin liquids (hot or cold meat can be used—skin and bones must be removed)
- Extremely Thick Stock— see recipe on page 55

DIRECTIONS

1. Add sauteed fish to food processor with sharp blade.
2. Put cover on processor.
3. Run processor for 15 seconds.
4. Open processor and evaluate fish for compliance with the size requirements for IDDSI ▼5 Minced & Moist:
   a. Remove any obviously burnt, extra crispy, undercooked, tough or stringy pieces.
   b. If all pieces are equal to or smaller than 4 mm x 4 mm x 15 mm, go to Step 5.
   c. If not, scrape all fish off the side of processor bowl and return to Step 2.
5. Put processed fish into a mixing bowl and stir with a spatula. Evaluate the moisture level, presence of water-thin liquid and cohesiveness:
   a. If water-thin liquid is visible in the bottom of the bowl or is separating from the fish, go to Step 6.
   b. If water-thin liquid is not visible and the fish appears dry and will not hold together, go to Step 6.
   c. If water-thin liquid is not present and the fish is moist and holds together, go to Step 7.
6. If water-thin liquid is present or the fish is too dry, it is necessary to add some ▲4 Thickened Stock to comply with IDDSI standards:
   a. Remove any excess thin liquid with a spoon.
   b. Add small amounts of ▲4 Thickened Stock to the fish and stir with spatula to thoroughly combine liquids and solids.
   c. Continue adding small amounts of ▲4 Extremely Thick Stock until fish is moist and no water-thin liquid is separating.
7. Evaluate to ensure compliance with IDDSI ▼5 Minced & Moist requirements:
   a. No separated water-thin liquids.
   b. Easily mashed with little pressure from a fork.
   c. Easily separates and comes through the tines of a fork.
   d. Holds its shape and slides off with little food left on a teaspoon.
8. Remove from bowl and serve, or separate into portions for storage.

Scrambled Eggs

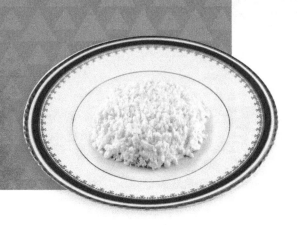

INGREDIENTS

- 4 eggs, scrambled and cooked (hot or cold)
- If necessary:
  - 1 oz. milk, slightly warmed to take the chill off
  - 1 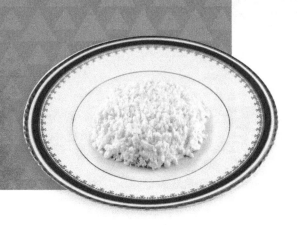 Mildly Thick packet (6g) or 1 pump stroke)

NOTES

Unused portions can be frozen and re-heated to serve. Typically, you will not need to add more liquid to scrambled eggs to meet IDDSI standards. However, it is common for scrambled eggs to "give up" water-thin liquids. Be prepared to drain water-thin liquids and monitor closely while eating to avoid choking risk.

DIRECTIONS

1. Add eggs to food processor with sharp blade.
2. Put cover on processor.
3. Run processor for 2–3 pulses.
4. Open processor and evaluate eggs for compliance with the size requirements for IDDSI 5 Minced & Moist:
   a. Remove any obviously burnt, overcooked, tough or stringy pieces.
   b. If all pieces are equal to or smaller than 4 mm x 4 mm x 15 mm, go to Step 5.
   c. If not, scrape side of processor bowl and return to Step 2.
5. Put processed eggs into a mixing bowl and stir with a spatula. Evaluate the moisture level, presence of water-thin liquid and cohesiveness:
   a. If water-thin liquid is visible in the bottom of the bowl or is separating from the eggs, go to Step 6.
   b. If water-thin liquid is not visible and the eggs appear dry and won't hold together, go to Step 6.
   c. If water-thin liquid is not present and the eggs are moist and hold together, go to Step 7.
6. If water-thin liquid is present or the eggs are too dry, it is necessary to add some milk thickened to 4 Extremely Thick to comply with IDDSI standards:
   a. Remove excess water-thin liquid with a spoon.
   b. Combine warmed milk with 6g SimplyThick® EasyMix™ and mix until thickened.
   c. Add small amounts of thickened milk to the eggs and stir with spatula to thoroughly combine liquids and solids.
   d. Continue adding small amounts of 4 Extremely Thick milk until eggs are moist and are able to hold together with no water-thin liquid separating.
7. Evaluate to ensure compliance with IDDSI 5 Minced & Moist requirements:
   a. No separated water-thin liquids.
   b. Easily mashed with little pressure from a fork.
   c. Easily separates and comes through the tines of a fork.
   d. Holds its shape and slides off with little food left on a teaspoon.
8. Remove from bowl and serve, or separate into portions for storage.

Egg Salad

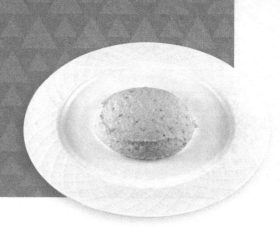

INGREDIENTS

- 16 oz. egg salad,* homemade or store-bought
- If necessary:
  - Mayonnaise

NOTES

Our testers found wide variations in the prepared egg salads found in stores. It is possible to process egg salad with a knife, however it can be tedious. We found the food processor to be quicker and more efficient.

We found that egg salad does not have ingredients that will be difficult to process. However, be on the lookout for celery, red and green peppers, or any nuts that would be difficult to process. Check the ingredient label to be certain. If you find an egg salad with these ingredients, it is easiest to manually remove them before processing. If you are following an egg salad recipe with these ingredients, simply omit them when you are making the egg salad. Egg salad may have red pimentos that look like red peppers, but these will process very easily.

DIRECTIONS

1. Add egg salad to a food processor with a sharp blade.
2. Put cover on processor.
3. Run processor for 5 seconds.
4. Open processor and evaluate egg salad for compliance with the size requirements for IDDSI ⑤ Minced & Moist:
   a. Remove any obviously undercooked, tough or stringy pieces.
   b. If all pieces are equal to or smaller than 4 mm x 4 mm x 15 mm, go to Step 8.
   c. If not, scrape all egg salad off the side of processor bowl and return to Step 7.
5. Put cover back on processor and process with 2–3 more 1-second bursts or pulses, depending on your processor. Return to Step 6.
6. Evaluate to ensure compliance with IDDSI ⑤ Minced & Moist requirements:
   a. No separated water-thin liquids.
   b. Easily mashed with little pressure from a fork.
   c. Easily separates and comes through the tines of a fork.
   d. Holds its shape and slides off with little food left on a teaspoon.
7. Remove from bowl and serve, or separate into portions for storage.

In our development and testing, we did not come across an egg salad that released water-thin liquids. We did not need to add any additional thick liquids to the egg salad when processing. If needed, add more mayonnaise to control any observed water-thin liquids present.

Potato Salad

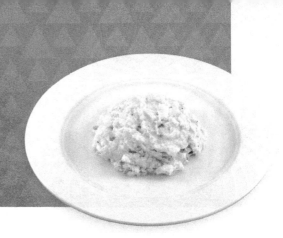

INGREDIENTS

- 16 oz. potato salad,* homemade or store-bought
- If necessary:
  - Mayonnaise

NOTES

We found that potato salad may not have ingredients that will be difficult to process. However, be on the lookout for celery, red and green peppers, or any nuts that would be difficult to process. Check the ingredient label to be certain. If you find a potato salad with these ingredients, it is easiest to manually remove them before processing. If you are following a potato salad recipe with these ingredients, simply omit them when you are making the potato salad.

DIRECTIONS

1. Add potato salad to a food processor with a sharp blade.
2. Put cover on processor.
3. Run processor for 5 seconds.
4. Open processor and evaluate potato salad for compliance with the size requirements for IDDSI 5 Minced & Moist:
   a. Remove any obviously undercooked, tough or stringy pieces.
   b. If all pieces are equal to or smaller than 4 mm x 4 mm x 15 mm, go to Step 8.
   c. If not, scrape all potato salad off the side of processor bowl and return to Step 7.
5. Put cover back on processor and process with 2–3 more 1-second bursts or pulses, depending on your processor. Return to Step 6.
6. Evaluate to ensure compliance with IDDSI 5 Minced & Moist requirements:
   a. No separated water-thin liquids.
   b. Easily mashed with little pressure from a fork.
   c. Easily separates and comes through the tines of a fork.
   d. Holds its shape and slides off with little food left on a teaspoon.
7. Remove from bowl and serve, or separate into portions for storage.

In our development and testing, we did not come across a potato salad that released water-thin liquids. We did not need to add any additional thick liquids to the potato salad when processing. If needed, add more mayonnaise to control any observed water-thin liquids present.

Chicken Salad

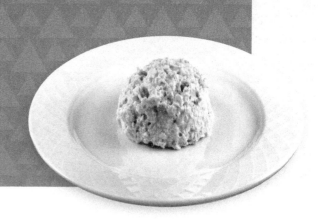

INGREDIENTS

- 16 oz. chicken salad,* homemade or store-bought
- If necessary:
  - Mayonnaise

NOTES

Our testers found wide variations in the prepared chicken salads found in stores. When possible, avoid purchasing chicken salad with ingredients that will make it difficult to process into ⑤ Minced & Moist. Avoid nuts, celery, raw peppers or any other difficult to process ingredient. However, due to the customary preparation, it is likely that you will not be able to avoid all of these ingredients. We recommend removing these pieces and cutting to the appropriate size with a kitchen knife. Then they may be incorporated back into the chicken salad, if appropriate for your diet. If you make chicken salad from scratch, we recommend cutting peppers and celery to the correct IDDSI size BEFORE adding to the recipe.

DIRECTIONS

1. Remove nuts, celery, red and green peppers larger than 4 mm.
2. Discard or use a knife to cut and chop until all pieces are smaller than 4 mm.
3. Add chicken salad and chopped celery, red and green peppers to food processor with a sharp blade.
4. Put cover on processor.
5. Run processor for 5 seconds.
6. Open processor and evaluate chicken salad for compliance with the size requirements for IDDSI ⑤ Minced & Moist:
   a. Remove any obviously undercooked, tough or stringy pieces.
   b. If all pieces are equal to or smaller than 4 mm x 4 mm x 15 mm, go to Step 8.
   c. If not, scrape all chicken salad off the side of processor bowl and return to Step 7.
7. Put cover back on processor and process with 2–3 more 1-second bursts or pulses, depending on your processor. Return to Step 6.
8. Evaluate to ensure compliance with IDDSI ⑤ Minced & Moist requirements:
   a. No separated water-thin liquids
   b. Easily mashed with little pressure from a fork.
   c. Easily separates and comes through the tines of a fork.
   d. Holds its shape and slides off with little food left on a teaspoon.
9. Remove from bowl and serve, or separate into portions for storage.

*In our development and testing, we did not come across a chicken salad that released water-thin liquids. We did not need to add any additional thick liquids to the chicken salad when processing. If needed, add more mayonnaise to control any observed water-thin liquids present.

Tuna Salad

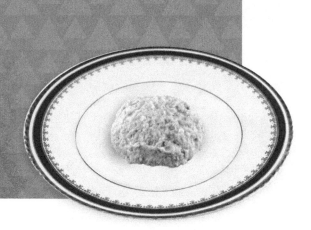

INGREDIENTS

- 16 oz. tuna salad,* homemade or store-bought
- If necessary:
  – Mayonnaise

NOTES

Our testers found wide variations in the prepared tuna salads found in stores. When possible, avoid purchasing tuna salad with ingredients that will make it difficult to process into 5 Minced & Moist. Avoid pine nuts, celery, raw peppers or any other difficult to process ingredient. However, due to the customary preparation, it is likely that you will not be able to avoid all of these ingredients. We recommend removing these pieces and cutting to the appropriate size with a kitchen knife. Then they may be incorporated back into the tuna salad, if appropriate for your diet. If you make tuna salad from scratch, we recommend cutting peppers and celery to the correct IDDSI size BEFORE adding to the recipe.

DIRECTIONS

1. Remove nuts, celery, red and green peppers larger than 4 mm.
2. Discard or use a knife to cut and chop until all pieces are smaller than 4 mm.
3. Add tuna salad and chopped celery, red and green peppers to food processor with a sharp blade.
4. Put cover on processor.
5. Run processor for 5 seconds.
6. Open processor and evaluate tuna salad for compliance with the size requirements for IDDSI 5 Minced & Moist:
   a. Remove any obviously undercooked, tough or stringy pieces.
   b. If all pieces are equal to or smaller than 4 mm x 4 mm x 15 mm, go to Step 8.
   c. If not, scrape all tuna salad off the side of processor bowl and return to Step 7.
7. Put cover back on processor and process with 2–3 more 1-second bursts or pulses, depending on your processor. Return to Step 6.
8. Evaluate to ensure compliance with IDDSI 5 Minced & Moist requirements:
   a. No separated water-thin liquids.
   b. Easily mashed with little pressure from a fork.
   c. Easily separates and comes through the tines of a fork.
   d. Holds its shape and slides off with little food left on a teaspoon.
9. Remove from bowl and serve, or separate into portions for storage.

*In our development and testing, we did not come across a tuna salad that released water-thin liquids. We did not need to add any additional thick liquids to the tuna salad when processing. If needed, add more mayonnaise to control any observed water-thin liquids present.

Coleslaw

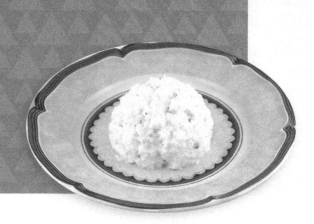

INGREDIENTS

- 16 oz. coleslaw, homemade or store-bought — drained of thin liquids
- 2–4 oz. mayonnaise, sour cream or 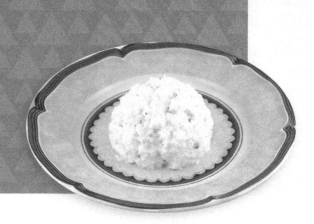 Extremely Thick Stock — see recipe on page 55

NOTES

Our testers used coleslaw from their local grocery stores. After processing the coleslaw there was often water-thin liquid present as cabbage release water as it is processed. Mayonnaise, sour cream, or ⚠ Extremely Thick Stock is added to hold these water-thin liquids in the slaw.

There are variations in the ingredient list for prepared coleslaw. When shopping, try to avoid products that have celery, pickles, pine nuts, or similar ingredients that will be tough to process. If these are present and difficult to process, they will have to be manually removed. If you make coleslaw from scratch, we recommend avoiding difficult to process ingredients.

DIRECTIONS

1. Add cooked coleslaw to a food processor with sharp blade.
2. Put cover on processor.
3. Run processor for 10 seconds.
4. Open processor and evaluate coleslaw for compliance with the size requirements for IDDSI ▽5 Minced & Moist:
   a. Remove any obviously tough or stringy pieces.
   b. If all pieces are equal to or smaller than 4 mm x 4 mm x 15 mm, go to Step 5.
   c. If not, scrape all coleslaw off the side of the processor bowl and return to Step 2.
5. Put processed coleslaw into a mixing bowl and stir with a spatula. Evaluate the moisture level and whether water-thin liquids are weeping or separating from the coleslaw:
   a. If water-thin liquid is visible in the bottom of the bowl or is separating from the coleslaw, go to Step 6.
   b. If water-thin liquid is not visible and the coleslaw appears dry and will not stick together, go to Step 6.
   c. If water-thin liquid is not present and the coleslaw is moist and holds together, go to Step 7.
6. If water-thin liquid is present or the coleslaw is too dry, it is necessary to add some mayonnaise, sour cream or ⚠ Extremely Thick Stock to the coleslaw to comply with IDDSI standards:
   a. If present, remove excess water-thin liquid with a spoon.
   b. Add small amounts of mayonnaise, sour cream or ⚠ Extremely Thick Stock to the coleslaw and stir with spatula to thoroughly combine liquids and solids.
   c. Continue adding small amounts of mayonnaise, sour cream or ⚠ Extremely Thick Stock until coleslaw is moist and no | water-thin liquid is separating.
7. Evaluate to ensure compliance with IDDSI ▽5 Minced & Moist requirements:
   a. No separated water-thin liquids.
   b. Easily mashed with little pressure from a fork.
   c. Easily separates and comes through the tines of a fork.
   d. Holds its shape and slides off with little food left on a teaspoon.
8. Remove from bowl and serve, or separate into portions for storage.

Carrots

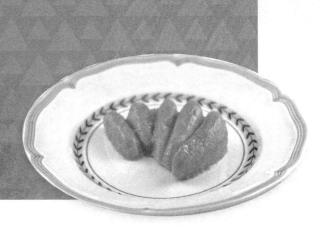

INGREDIENTS

- 2 cups (16 oz.) carrots cooked until tender enough to be pierced or cut easily with a fork (hot or cold)
- Extremely Thick Stock— see recipe on page 55

NOTES

This process will work with both hot and cold cooked carrots. The amount of Extremely Thick Stock needed will vary depending on whether you are using canned, frozen, or fresh carrots. Canned carrots, even after draining, brought significantly more water-thin liquid with them and required more Extremely Thick Stock to control the water-thin liquids present. On occasion no Extremely Thick Stock is required to achieve the perfect Minced & Moist texture. Rely on the process and your test results to ensure proper preparation.

DIRECTIONS

1. Add carrots to a food processor with sharp blade.
2. Put cover on processor.
3. Run processor for 10 seconds.
4. Open processor and evaluate carrots for compliance with the size requirements for IDDSI 5 Minced & Moist:
   a. Remove any obviously undercooked, tough or stringy pieces.
   b. If all pieces are equal to or smaller than 4 mm x 4 mm x 15 mm, go to Step 5.
   c. If not, scrape all carrots off the side of the processor bowl and return to Step 2.
5. Put processed carrots into a mixing bowl and stir with a spatula. Evaluate the moisture level and whether water-thin liquids are weeping or separating from the carrots:
   a. If water-thin liquid is visible in the bottom of the bowl or is separating from the carrots, go to Step 6.
   b. If water-thin liquid is not visible and the carrots appears dry and will not stick together, go to Step 6.
   c. If water-thin liquid is not present and the carrots are moist and hold together, go to Step 7.
6. If water-thin liquid is present or the carrots are too dry, it is necessary to add some Extremely Thick Stock to the carrots to comply with IDDSI standards:
   a. If excess water-thin liquids are present, remove with a spoon.
   b. Add small amounts of Extremely Thick Stock to the carrots and stir with spatula to thoroughly combine liquids and solids.
   c. Continue adding small amounts of Extremely Thick Stock until carrots are moist and no water-thin liquid is separating.
7. Evaluate to ensure compliance with IDDSI 5 Minced & Moist requirements:
   a. No separated water-thin liquids.
   b. Easily mashed with little pressure from a fork.
   c. Easily separates and comes through the tines of a fork.
   d. Holds its shape and slides off with little food left on a teaspoon.
8. Remove from bowl and serve, or separate into portions for storage.

Cauliflower

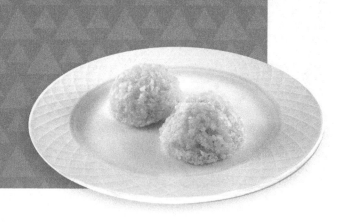

INGREDIENTS

- 2 cups (16 oz.) cauliflower cooked until tender enough to be pierced or cut easily with a fork (hot or cold)
- Extremely Thick Stock— see recipe on page 55

NOTES

This process will work with both hot and cold cooked cauliflower. The total amount of 4 Extremely Thick Stock needed will vary based on whether you start with frozen or fresh cauliflower, and whether you cook it in the microwave or by steaming. Cooking cauliflower to well done will reduce the processing time. With cauliflower, you may find that no additional 4 Extremely Thick Stock is required to process properly. Rely on the process and your test results to ensure proper preparation.

DIRECTIONS

1. Add cauliflower to a food processor with sharp blade.
2. Put cover on processor.
3. Run processor for 10 seconds.
4. Open processor and evaluate cauliflower for compliance with the size requirements for IDDSI 5 Minced & Moist:
   a. Remove any obviously undercooked, tough or stringy pieces.
   b. If all pieces are equal to or smaller than 4 mm x 4 mm x 15 mm, go to Step 5.
   c. If not, scrape all cauliflower off the side of the processor bowl and return to Step 2.
5. Put processed cauliflower into a mixing bowl and stir with a spatula. Evaluate the moisture level and whether water-thin liquids are weeping or separating from the cauliflower:
   a. If water-thin liquid is visible in the bottom of the bowl or is separating from the cauliflower, go to Step 6.
   b. If water-thin liquid is not visible and the cauliflower appears dry and will not stick together, go to Step 6.
   c. If water-thin liquid is not present and the cauliflower is moist and holds together, go to Step 7.
6. If water-thin liquid is present or the cauliflower is too dry, it is necessary to add some 4 Extremely Thick Stock to the cauliflower to comply with IDDSI standards:
   a. If excess water-thin liquids are present, remove with a spoon.
   b. Add small amounts of 4 Extremely Thick Stock to the cauliflower and stir with spatula to thoroughly combine liquids and solids.
   c. Continue adding small amounts of 4 Extremely Thick Stock until cauliflower is moist and no water-thin liquid is separating.
7. Evaluate to ensure compliance with IDDSI 5 Minced & Moist requirements:
   a. No separated water-thin liquids.
   b. Easily mashed with little pressure from a fork.
   c. Easily separates and comes through the tines of a fork.
   d. Holds its shape and slides off with little food left on a teaspoon.
8. Remove from bowl and serve, or separate into portions for storage.

Broccoli

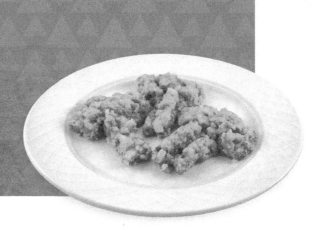

INGREDIENTS

- 2 cups (16 oz.) broccoli cooked until the thicker stems are tender enough to be pierced or cut easily with a fork (hot or cold)
- Extremely Thick Stock— see recipe on page 55

NOTES

This process will work with both hot or cold cooked broccoli. Due to the natural moisture content of broccoli, the use of Extremely Thick Stock is rarely needed.

DIRECTIONS

1. Add cooked broccoli to a food processor with sharp blade.
2. Put cover on processor.
3. Run processor for 10 seconds.
4. Open processor and evaluate broccoli for compliance with the size requirements for IDDSI 5 Minced & Moist:
   a. Remove any obviously undercooked, tough or stringy pieces.
   b. If all pieces are equal to or smaller than 4 mm x 4 mm x 15 mm, go to Step 5.
   c. If not, scrape all broccoli off the side of the processor bowl and return to Step 2.
5. Put processed broccoli into a mixing bowl and stir with a spatula. Evaluate the moisture level and whether water-thin liquids are weeping or separating from the broccoli:
   a. If water-thin liquid is visible in the bottom of the bowl or is separating from the broccoli, go to Step 6.
   b. If water-thin liquid is not visible and the broccoli appears dry and will not stick together, go to Step 6.
   c. If water-thin liquid is not present and the broccoli is moist and holds together, go to Step 7.
6. If water-thin liquid is present or the broccoli is too dry, it is necessary to add some 4 Extremely Thick Stock to the broccoli to comply with IDDSI standards:
   a. If excess water-thin liquids are present, remove with a spoon.
   b. Add small amounts of 4 Extremely Thick Stock to the broccoli and stir with spatula to thoroughly combine liquids and solids.
   c. Continue adding small amounts of 4 Extremely Thick Stock until broccoli is moist and no water-thin liquid is separating.
7. Evaluate to ensure compliance with IDDSI 5 Minced & Moist requirements:
   a. No separated water-thin liquids.
   b. Easily mashed with little pressure from a fork.
   c. Easily separates and comes through the tines of a fork.
   d. Holds its shape and slides off with little food left on a teaspoon.
8. Remove from bowl and serve, or separate into portions for storage.

Bonus presentation tip: Put 5 Minced & Moist broccoli into a pastry bag with tip or zip-style plastic bag. Use a pastry tip or cut off a corner of the bag to pipe onto plate for improved presentation.

Butternut Squash

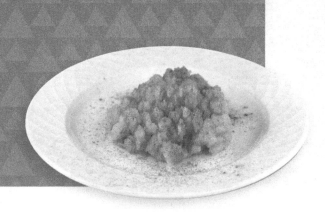

INGREDIENTS

- 2 cups (16 oz.) butternut squash cooked until tender enough to be pierced or cut easily with a fork and drained thoroughly (hot or cold)
- 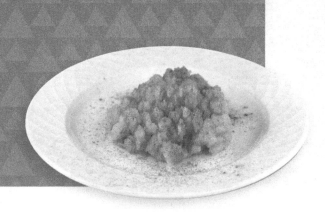 Extremely Thick Stock— see recipe on page 55

NOTES

This process will work with both hot or cold butternut squash.

The ripeness, moistness and softness of the particular butternut squash you are processing will impact the amount of ④ Extremely Thick Stock needed. With some butternut squashes, you may find that no additional ④ Extremely Thick Stock is required to process properly. Rely on the process and your test results to ensure proper preparation.

DIRECTIONS

1. Add cooked butternut squash to a food processor with sharp blade.
2. Put cover on processor.
3. Run processor for 10 seconds.
4. Open processor and evaluate butternut squash for compliance with the size requirements for IDDSI ⑤ Minced & Moist:
    a. Remove any obviously undercooked, tough or stringy pieces.
    b. If all pieces are equal to or smaller than 4 mm x 4 mm x 15 mm, go to Step 5.
    c. If not, scrape all butternut squash off the side of the processor bowl and return to Step 2.
5. Put processed butternut squash into a mixing bowl and stir with a spatula. Evaluate the moisture level and whether water-thin liquids are weeping or separating from the butternut squash:
    a. If water-thin liquid is visible in the bottom of the bowl or is separating from the butternut squash, go to Step 6.
    b. If water-thin liquid is not visible and the butternut squash appears dry and will not stick together, go to Step 6.
    c. If water-thin liquid is not present and the butternut squash is moist and holds together, go to Step 7.
6. If water-thin liquid is present or the butternut squash is too dry, it is necessary to add some ④ Extremely Thick Stock to the butternut squash to comply with IDDSI standards:
    a. If excess water-thin liquids are present, remove with a spoon.
    b. Add small amounts of ④ Extremely Thick Stock to the butternut squash and stir with spatula to thoroughly combine liquids and solids.
    c. Continue adding small amounts ④ Extremely Thick Stock until butternut squash is moist and no water-thin liquid is separating.
7. Evaluate to ensure compliance with IDDSI ⑤ Minced & Moist requirements:
    a. No separated water-thin liquids.
    b. Easily mashed with little pressure from a fork.
    c. Easily separates and comes through the tines of a fork.
    d. Holds its shape and slides off with little food left on a teaspoon.
8. Remove from bowl and serve, or separate into portions for storage.

Bonus presentation tip: Sprinkle with cinnamon (if approved by your SLP).

MINCED & MOIST

Green Beans

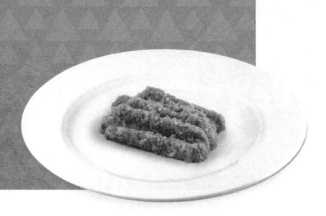

INGREDIENTS

- 2 cups (16 oz.) green beans cooked until tender enough to be pierced or cut easily with a fork, drained of all drippings and thin liquids (hot or cold)
- ▲ Extremely Thick Stock— see recipe on page 55

NOTES

This process will work with both hot and cold cooked green beans. The amount of ▲ Extremely Thick Stock needed will vary based on whether you are using canned, frozen, or fresh green beans. Even after draining, canned beans brought significantly more thin liquid into the food processor and required more ▲ Extremely Thick Stock. Most of the time, no ▲ Extremely Thick Stock is required to achieve the perfect ▽ Minced & Moist texture. Rely on the process and your test results to ensure proper preparation.

DIRECTIONS

1. Add green beans to a food processor with sharp blade.
2. Put cover on processor.
3. Run processor for 10 seconds.
4. Open processor and evaluate green beans for compliance with the size requirements for IDDSI ▽ Minced & Moist:
   a. Remove any obviously undercooked, tough or stringy pieces.
   b. If all pieces are equal to or smaller than 4 mm x 4 mm x 15 mm, go to Step 5.
   c. If not, scrape all green beans off the side of the processor bowl and return to Step 2.
5. Put processed green beans into a mixing bowl and stir with a spatula. Evaluate the moisture level and whether water-thin liquids are weeping or separating from the green beans:
   a. If water-thin liquid is visible in the bottom of the bowl or is separating from the green beans, go to Step 6.
   b. If water-thin liquid is not visible and the green beans appear dry and will not stick together, go to Step 6.
   c. If water-thin liquid is not present and the green beans are moist and hold together, go to Step 7.
6. If water-thin liquid is present or the green beans are too dry, it is necessary to add some ▲ Extremely Thick Stock to the green beans to comply with IDDSI standards:
   a. If excess water-thin liquids are present, remove with a spoon.
   b. Add small amounts of ▲ Extremely Thick Stock to the green beans and stir with spatula to thoroughly combine liquids and solids.
   c. Continue adding small amounts of ▲ Extremely Thick Stock until green beans are moist and no water-thin liquid is separating.
7. Evaluate to ensure compliance with IDDSI ▽ Minced & Moist requirements:
   a. No separated water-thin liquids.
   b. Easily mashed with little pressure from a fork.
   c. Easily separates and comes through the tines of a fork.
   d. Holds its shape and slides off with little food left on a teaspoon.
8. Remove from bowl and serve, or separate into portions for storage.

Peas

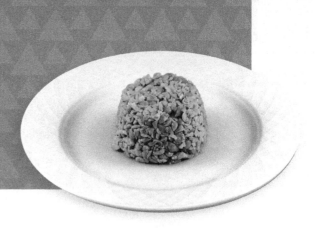

INGREDIENTS

- 2 cups (16 oz.) peas cooked until tender enough to be pierced or cut easily with a fork and drained thoroughly (hot or cold)
- 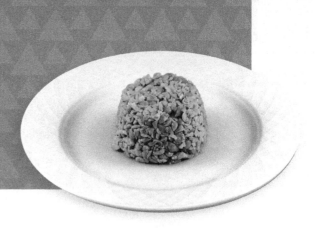 Extremely Thick Stock— see recipe on page 55

NOTES

This process will work with both hot or cold peas. The amount of ▲ Extremely Thick Stock needed will vary depending on whether you are starting with frozen, canned or fresh peas. Canned peas, even after draining, simply have significantly more water-thin liquid within them and will usually require more ▲ Extremely Thick Stock to control the water-thin liquids present. On occasion no ▲ Extremely Thick Stock is required to achieve the perfect ▼ Minced & Moist texture. Rely on the process and your test results to ensure proper preparation.

DIRECTIONS

1. Add cooked peas to a food processor with sharp blade.
2. Put cover on processor.
3. Run processor for 2–3 seconds.
4. Open processor and evaluate peas for compliance with the size requirements for IDDSI ▼ Minced & Moist:
   a. Remove any obviously undercooked, tough or stringy pieces.
   b. If all pieces are equal to or smaller than 4 mm x 4 mm x 15 mm, go to Step 5.
   c. If not, scrape all peas off the side of the processor bowl and return to Step 2.
5. Put processed peas into a mixing bowl and stir with a spatula. Evaluate the moisture level and whether water-thin liquids are weeping or separating from the peas:
   a. If water-thin liquid is visible in the bottom of the bowl or is separating from the peas, go to Step 6.
   b. If water-thin liquid is not visible and the peas appear dry and will not stick together, go to Step 6.
   c. If water-thin liquid is not present and the peas are moist and hold together, go to Step 7.
6. If water-thin liquid is present or the peas are too dry, it is necessary to add some ▲ Extremely Thick Stock to the peas to comply with IDDSI standards:
   a. If excess water-thin liquids are present, remove with a spoon.
   b. Add small amounts of ▲ Extremely Thick Stock to the peas and stir with spatula to thoroughly combine liquids and solids.
   c. Continue adding small amounts of ▲ Extremely Thick Stock until the peas are moist and no water-thin liquid is separating.
7. Evaluate to ensure compliance with IDDSI ▼ Minced & Moist requirements:
   a. No separated water-thin liquids.
   b. Easily mashed with little pressure from a fork.
   c. Easily separates and comes through the tines of a fork.
   d. Holds its shape and slides off with little food left on a teaspoon.
8. Remove from bowl and serve, or separate into portions for storage.

Snow or Sugar Snap Peas

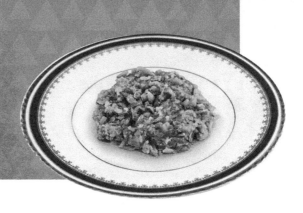

INGREDIENTS

- 2 cups (16 oz.) snow peas or sugar snap peas cooked in the pod until tender enough to be pierced or cut easily with a fork and drained thoroughly (hot or cold)
- ▲ Extremely Thick Stock— see recipe on page 55

NOTES

Snow and sugar snap are cooked and processed in their pods and can be successfully processed to ▽ Minced & Moist. However, they are too stringy to be successfully processed to ▽ Pureed.

DIRECTIONS

1. Add cooked peas to a food processor with sharp blade.
2. Put cover on processor.
3. Run processor for 10 seconds.
4. Open processor and evaluate peas for compliance with the size requirements for IDDSI ▽ Minced & Moist:
   a. Remove any obviously undercooked, tough or stringy pieces.
   b. If all pieces are equal to or smaller than 4 mm x 4 mm x 15 mm, go to Step 5.
   c. If not, scrape all peas off the side of the processor bowl and return to Step 2.
5. Put processed peas into a mixing bowl and stir with a spatula. Evaluate the moisture level and whether water-thin liquids are weeping or separating from the peas:
   a. If water-thin liquid is visible in the bottom of the bowl or is separating from the peas, go to Step 6.
   b. If water-thin liquid is not visible and the peas appear dry and will not stick together, go to Step 6.
   c. If water-thin liquid is not present and the peas are moist and hold together, go to Step 7.
6. If water-thin liquid is present or the peas are too dry, it is necessary to add some ▲ Extremely Thick Stock to the peas to comply with IDDSI standards:
   a. If excess water-thin liquids are present, remove with a spoon.
   b. Add small amounts of ▲ Extremely Thick Stock to the peas and stir with spatula to thoroughly combine liquids and solids.
   c. Continue adding small amounts of ▲ Extremely Thick Stock until peas are moist and no water-thin liquid is separating.
7. Evaluate to ensure compliance with IDDSI ▽ Minced & Moist requirements:
   a. No separated water-thin liquids.
   b. Easily mashed with little pressure from a fork.
   c. Easily separates and comes through the tines of a fork.
   d. Holds its shape and slides off with little food left on a teaspoon.
8. Remove from bowl and serve, or separate into portions for storage.

Spinach

INGREDIENTS

- 2 cups (16 oz.) spinach cooked until tender enough to be cut easily with a fork and drained thoroughly (hot or cold)
- ⚠ Extremely Thick Stock— see recipe on page 55

NOTES

This process will work with both hot and cold cooked spinach. Most of the time, you will NOT need to add any ⚠ Extremely Thick Stock to cooked spinach. Rely on the process and your test results to ensure proper preparation.

DIRECTIONS

1. Add cooked spinach to a food processor with sharp blade.
2. Put cover on processor.
3. Run processor for 10 seconds.
4. Open processor and evaluate spinach for compliance with the size requirements for IDDSI ▽5 Minced & Moist:
   a. Remove any obviously undercooked, tough or stringy pieces.
   b. If all pieces are equal to or smaller than 4 mm x 4 mm x 15 mm, go to Step 5.
   c. If not, scrape all spinach off the side of the processor bowl and return to Step 2.
5. Put processed spinach into a mixing bowl and stir with a spatula. Evaluate the moisture level and whether water-thin liquids are weeping or separating from the spinach:
   a. If water-thin liquid is visible in the bottom of the bowl or is separating from the spinach, go to Step 6.
   b. If water-thin liquid is not visible and the spinach appears dry and will not stick together, go to Step 6.
   c. If water-thin liquid is not present and the spinach is moist and holds together, go to Step 7.
6. If water-thin liquid is present or the spinach is too dry, it is necessary to add some ⚠ Extremely Thick Stock to the spinach to comply with IDDSI standards:
   a. If excess water-thin liquids are present, remove with a spoon.
   b. Add small amounts of ⚠ Extremely Thick Stock to the spinach and stir with spatula to thoroughly combine liquids and solids.
   c. Continue adding small amounts of ⚠ Extremely Thick Stock until spinach is moist and no water-thin liquid is separating.
7. Evaluate to ensure compliance with IDDSI ▽5 Minced & Moist requirements:
   a. No separated water-thin liquids.
   b. Easily mashed with little pressure from a fork.
   c. Easily separates and comes through the tines of a fork.
   d. Holds its shape and slides off with little food left on a teaspoon.
8. Remove from bowl and serve, or separate into portions for storage.

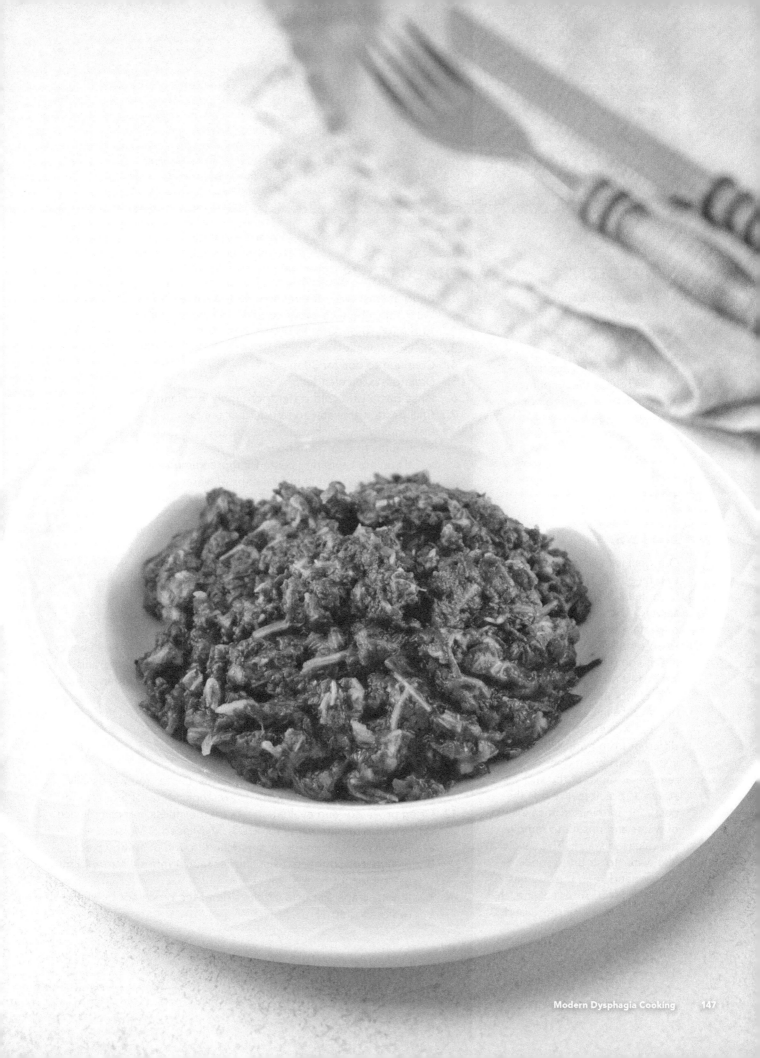

Buttered Noodles

INGREDIENTS

- 4 oz. (approx. 1 cup) dry pasta (elbow macaroni or angel hair/thin spaghetti are recommended)
- Water for boiling noodles — at least twice the amount recommended on the box
- 2 cups or more water for water bath
- Ice (optional)
- 4 oz. milk
- 2 tablespoons butter

NOTES

Our goal is to provide recipes that meet the IDDSI standards for at least 30 minutes after serving. The inherent starchiness of pasta made this a challenge to accomplish. In our quest for IDDSI-compliant pasta dishes, we tested pasta with a variety of cooking times—from al dente to falling apart. The process we settled upon is a bit different from traditional pasta instructions, but it does reliably remove as much of the sticky starch as possible. We boil the pasta for 30 minutes in an excess of water and rinse it to remove the released starch. Then, we chill it in water to stop the cooking process and keep the noodles moist and soft. After cooling, the pasta is ready to be processed and re-heated.

DIRECTIONS

1. Bring at least twice the recommended amount of water to a boil. We want to be sure every noodle is able to be fully cooked.
2. Add pasta and return to boil.
3. Stir occasionally.
4. Continue to boil for 30 minutes.
5. Drain pasta in colander.
6. Rinse pasta with cold water thoroughly in colander.
7. Chill pasta with water to refrigerator temperature—at or below 40°F (depending on which technique you use, this will take at least 30 minutes to 8 or more hours):
   a. If you are preparing pasta for more immediate use:
      i. Add ice and at least 4 cups of water to a large mixing bowl.
      ii. Add hot, drained, and rinsed pasta to ice water and mixing bowl.
      iii. Ensure the water level covers the pasta to chill and keep moist.
      iv. If hot pasta melts all the ice, add more ice to the bowl.
      v. Let pasta cool for at least 30 minutes.
   b. If you are preparing pasta for future use:
      i. Add hot, drained and rinsed pasta to an air-tight container or zip-style plastic bag.
      ii. Add enough water to ensure the pasta is covered in water. The amount will vary based on your container size and shape, but it will likely be 2 or more cups of water.
      iii. Put in refrigerator for at least 8 hours.
      iv. Use within 2 days.
8. When ready to serve, drain cooled pasta in colander.
9. Add pasta, milk and butter to food processor with a sharp blade.
10. Put cover on processor.
11. Run processor 5 times in 1-second pulses. (Note: You will usually need to cycle through these next few steps a total of 5 or 6 times.)
12. Open processor and evaluate pasta for moistness and compliance with the size requirements for IDDSI 5 Minced & Moist:
    a. Remove any obviously undercooked, tough or stringy pieces.
    b. If all pieces are equal to or smaller than 4 mm x 4 mm x 15 mm, go to Step 12.
    c. If not, scrape all pasta off the side of the processor bowl and return to Step 11.

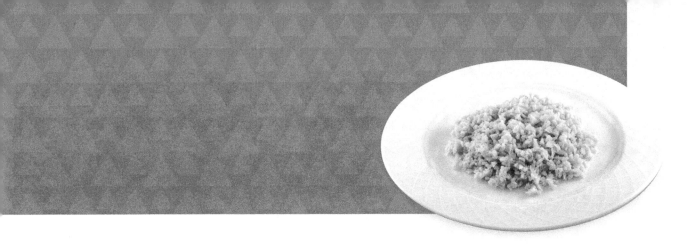

13. Evaluate to ensure compliance with IDDSI ⑤ Minced & Moist requirements:
    a. No separated water-thin liquids.
    b. Easily mashed with little pressure from a fork.
    c. Easily separates and comes through the tines of a fork.
    d. Holds its shape and slides off with little food left on a teaspoon.
14. If pasta is too sticky to pass IDDSI ⑤ Minced & Moist requirements, add a little additional milk or butter and return to Step 10.
15. Remove from bowl and separate into portions for storage or serving.
16. When serving, add noodles to a pastry bag with a round tip in place. Or simply add to a plastic bag and snip one corner off the bag. Pipe onto serving dish to give the appearance of noodles.
17. Use microwave or steamer (basket) to bring to serving temperature.

Homemade Shells & Cheese

INGREDIENTS

- 4 oz. dry shell pasta
- 4 oz. Velveeta® Original pasteurized recipe cheese product
- Water for boiling noodles— at least twice the amount recommended on the box
- 2 cups or more water for water bath
- Ice (optional)
- 2 oz. milk

NOTES

Our goal is to provide recipes that meet the IDDSI standards for at least 30 minutes after serving. The inherent starchiness of pasta made this a challenge to accomplish. In our quest for IDDSI-compliant pasta dishes, we tested pasta with a variety of cooking times—from al dente to falling apart. The process we settled upon is a bit different from traditional pasta instructions, but it does reliably remove as much of the sticky starch as possible. We boil the pasta for 30 minutes in an excess of water and rinse it to remove the released starch. Then, we chill it in water to stop the cooking process and keep the noodles moist and soft. After cooling, the pasta is ready to be processed and re-heated.

DIRECTIONS

1. Bring at least twice the package recommended amount of water to a boil. The goal is to be sure every noodle is able to be fully cooked.
2. Add pasta and return to boil.
3. Stir occasionally.
4. Continue to boil for 30 minutes.
5. Drain pasta in colander.
6. Rinse pasta with cold water thoroughly in colander.
7. Chill pasta with water to refrigerator temperature—at or below 40°F (depending on which technique you use, this will take at least 30 minutes to 8 or more hours):
   a. If you are preparing pasta for more immediate use:
      i. Add ice and at least 4 cups of water to a large mixing bowl.
      ii. Add hot, drained, and rinsed pasta to ice water and mixing bowl.
      iii. Ensure the water level covers the pasta to chill and keep moist.
      iv. If hot pasta melts all the ice, add more ice to the bowl.
      v. Let pasta cool for at least 30 minutes.
   b. If you are preparing pasta for future use:
      i. Add hot, drained and rinsed pasta to an air-tight container or zip-style plastic bag.
      ii. Add enough water to ensure the pasta is covered in water. The amount will vary based on your container size and shape, but it will likely be 2 or more cups of water.
      iii. Put in refrigerator for at least 8 hours.
      iv. Use within 2 days.
8. When ready to serve, drain cooled pasta in colander.
9. Add pasta, milk and Velveeta® Original cheese product to food processor with a sharp blade.
10. Put cover on processor.
11. Run processor 5 times in 1-second pulses. (Note: You will usually need to cycle through these next few steps a total of 5 or 6 times.)
12. Open processor and evaluate pasta for compliance with the size requirements for IDDSI 5 Minced & Moist:
    a. Remove any obviously undercooked, tough or stringy pieces.
    b. If all pieces are equal to or smaller than 4 mm x 4 mm x 15 mm, go to Step 12.
    c. If not, scrape all pasta off the side of the processor bowl and return to Step 11.

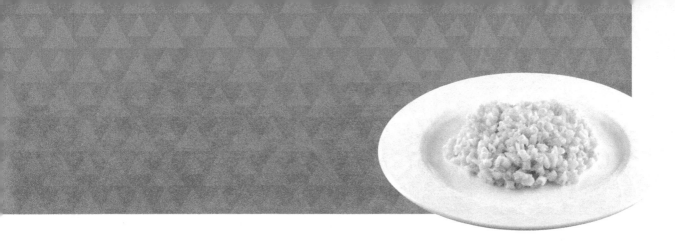

13. Using this process, you may reach the size requirements of ▽5 Minced & Moist before the cheese is completely blended into the pasta. Rather than continuing to decrease the noodle size in the food processor, add the contents of the processor bowl to a microwave safe bowl. Mix with a spatula until well blended. If needed, microwave for 5–10 seconds to help smooth out cheese.

14. Evaluate to ensure compliance with IDDSI ▽5 Minced & Moist requirements:
    a. No separated water-thin liquids.
    b. Easily mashed with little pressure from a fork.
    c. Easily separates and comes through the tines of a fork.
    d. Holds its shape and slides off with little food left on a teaspoon.

15. Remove from bowl and separate into portions for storage or serving.

16. When serving, add noodles to a pastry bag with a round tip in place. Or simply add to a plastic bag and snip one corner off the bag. Pipe onto serving dish to give the appearance of noodles.

17. Use microwave or steamer (basket) to bring to serving temperature.

Velveeta® Shells & Cheese Original

INGREDIENTS

- 1 box Velveeta® Shells & Cheese—Original (12 oz.) (Each box contains shells and 1 liquid gold cheese sauce pouch)
- 12 cups water for boiling noodles
- 2 cups or more water for water bath
- Ice (optional)
- 2 oz. milk

NOTES

The "Liquid Gold" cheese sauce supplied in the box is very helpful in processing this dish because it is a ④ Extremely Thick liquid at room temperature.

Read "Notes" on the following page before proceeding.

DIRECTIONS

1. Bring water to a boil in a large pot.
2. Add pasta and return to boil.
3. Stir occasionally.
4. Continue to boil for 30 minutes.
5. Drain pasta in colander.
6. Rinse pasta with cold water thoroughly in colander.
7. Chill pasta with water to refrigerator temperature—at or below 40°F (depending on which technique you use, this will take at least 30 minutes to 8 or more hours):
   a. If you are preparing pasta for more immediate use:
      i. Add ice and at least 4 cups of water to a large mixing bowl.
      ii. Add hot, drained, and rinsed pasta to ice water and mixing bowl.
      iii. Ensure the water level covers the pasta to chill and keep moist.
      iv. If hot pasta melts all the ice, add more ice to the bowl.
      v. Let pasta cool for at least 30 minutes.
   b. If you are preparing pasta for future use:
      i. Add hot, drained and rinsed pasta to an air-tight container or zip-style plastic bag.
      ii. Add enough water to ensure the pasta is covered in water. The amount will vary based on your container size and shape, but it will likely be 2 or more cups of water.
      iii. Put in refrigerator for at least 8 hours.
      iv. Use within 2 days.
8. When ready to serve, drain cooled pasta in colander.
9. Add pasta, milk and Liquid Gold cheese sauce pouch to food processor with a sharp blade.
10. Put cover on processor.
11. Run processor 5 times in 1-second pulses. (Note: You will usually need to cycle through these next few steps a total of 5 or 6 times.)
12. Open processor and evaluate pasta for compliance with the size requirements for IDDSI ▽5 Minced & Moist:
    a. Remove any obviously undercooked, tough or stringy pieces.
    b. If all pieces are equal to or smaller than 4 mm x 4 mm x 15 mm, go to Step 12.
    c. If not, scrape all pasta off the side of the processor bowl and return to Step 11.

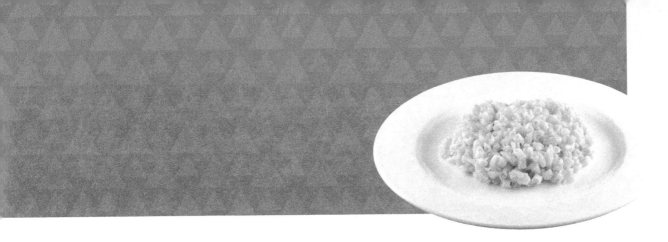

13. Using this process, you may reach the size requirements of ▼5 Minced & Moist before the cheese sauce is completely blended into the pasta. Rather than continuing to decrease the noodle size in the food processor, add the contents of the processor bowl to a microwave safe bowl. Mix with a spatula until well blended.
14. Evaluate to ensure compliance with IDDSI ▼5 Minced & Moist requirements:
    a. No separated water-thin liquids.
    b. Easily mashed with little pressure from a fork.
    c. Easily separates and comes through the tines of a fork.
    d. Holds its shape and slides off with little food left on a teaspoon.
15. Remove from bowl and separate into portions for storage or serving.
16. When serving, add noodles to a pastry bag with a round tip in place. Or simply add to a plastic bag and snip one corner off the bag. Pipe onto serving dish to give the appearance of noodles.
17. Use microwave or steamer (basket) to bring to serving temperature.

NOTES

Our goal is to provide recipes that meet the IDDSI standards for at least 30 minutes after serving. The inherent starchiness of pasta made this a challenge to accomplish. In our quest for IDDSI-compliant pasta dishes, we tested pasta with a variety of cooking times—from al dente to falling apart. The process we settled upon is a bit different from traditional pasta instructions, but it does reliably remove as much of the sticky starch as possible. We boil the pasta for 30 minutes in an excess of water and rinse it to remove the released starch. Then, we chill it in water to stop the cooking process and keep the noodles moist and soft. After cooling, the pasta is ready to be processed and re-heated.

Spaghetti & Meatballs

INGREDIENTS

- 4 oz. (approx. 1 cup) dry pasta (elbow macaroni or angel hair/thin spaghetti are recommended)
- Water for boiling noodles—at least twice the amount recommended on the box
- 2 cups or more water for water bath
- Ice (optional)
- 4 oz. milk
- 16 oz. ⓐ Extremely Thick Marinara Sauce—see recipe on page 54
- 12–16 oz. 5 Minced & Moist Meatballs—see recipe on page 124 (optional)

NOTES

This recipe is a capstone in our learning to process our favorite foods into IDDSI-compliant dishes. We combine the processing of up to 3 separate components to produce a wonderful, tasty meal. Because of the time required to process the pasta, you will have time to make the sauce and the optional meatballs while the noodles are cooking and cooling.

Read "Notes" on the following page before proceeding.

DIRECTIONS

1. Bring at least twice the recommended amount of water to a boil. We want to be sure every noodle is able to be fully cooked.
2. Add pasta and return to boil.
3. Stir occasionally.
4. Continue to boil for 30 minutes.

While pasta is cooking prepare ⓐ Extremely Thick Marinara Sauce and (optional) 5 Minced & Moist Meatballs.

5. Drain pasta in colander.
6. Rinse pasta with cold water thoroughly in colander.
7. Chill pasta with water to refrigerator temperature—at or below 40°F (depending on which technique you use, this will take at least 30 minutes to 8 or more hours):
   a. If you are preparing pasta for more immediate use:
      i. Add ice and at least 4 cups of water to a large mixing bowl.
      ii. Add hot, drained, and rinsed pasta to ice water and mixing bowl.
      iii. Ensure the water level covers the pasta to chill and keep moist.
      iv. If hot pasta melts all the ice, add more ice to the bowl.
      v. Let pasta cool for at least 30 minutes.
   b. If you are preparing pasta for future use:
      i. Add hot, drained and rinsed pasta to an air-tight container or zip-style plastic bag.
      ii. Add enough water to ensure the pasta is covered in water. The amount will vary based on your container size and shape, but it will likely be 2 or more cups of water.
      iii. Put in refrigerator for at least 8 hours.
      iv. Use within 2 days.
8. When ready to serve, drain cooled pasta in colander.
9. Add pasta and HALF of the milk to food processor with a sharp blade.
10. Put cover on processor.
11. Run processor 5 times in 1-second pulses. (Note: you will usually need to cycle through these next few steps a total of 5 or 6 times.)

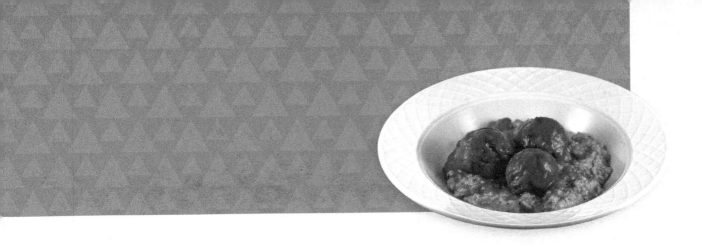

12. Open processor and evaluate pasta for moistness and compliance with the size requirements for IDDSI ⑤ Minced & Moist:
    a. Remove any obviously undercooked, tough or stringy pieces.
    b. If pasta needs more moisture, add a little more milk and return to Step 9.
    c. If all pieces are equal to or smaller than 4 mm x 4 mm x 15 mm, go to Step 12.
    d. If not, scrape all pasta off the side of the processor bowl and return to Step 9.
13. Evaluate to ensure compliance with IDDSI ⑤ Minced & Moist requirements:
    a. No separated water-thin liquids.
    b. Easily mashed with little pressure from a fork.
    c. Easily separates and comes through the tines of a fork.
    d. Holds its shape and slides off with little food left on a teaspoon.
14. If pasta is too sticky to passes IDDSI ⑤ Minced & Moist requirements, add a little additional milk and return to Step 10.
15. At this point, you have the option to choose how you would like to serve the dish:
    a. For sauce premixed with the noodles:
        i. Add pasta to a mixing bowl and add ④ Extremely Thick Marinara Sauce to taste.
        ii. Mix with spatula until well blended.
        iii. Add pasta and sauce to a pastry bag with a round tip in place. Or, simply add to a plastic bag and snip one corner off the bag. Pipe onto serving dish to give the appearance of noodles mixed with sauce.
        iv. [Optional] Top with meatballs.
    b. For sauce on top presentation:
        i. Add pasta to a pastry bag with a round tip in place. Or simply add to a plastic bag and snip one corner off the bag. Pipe onto serving dish to give the appearance of noodles.
        ii. Top with ④ Extremely Thick Marinara Sauce.
        iii. [Optional] Top with meatballs.
15. Use microwave to bring to serving temperature.

NOTES

Our goal is to provide recipes that meet the IDDSI standards for at least 30 minutes after serving. The inherent starchiness of pasta made this a challenge to accomplish. In our quest for IDDSI-compliant pasta dishes, we tested pasta with a variety of cooking times—from al dente to falling apart. The process we settled upon is a bit different from traditional pasta instructions, but it does reliably remove as much of the sticky starch as possible. We boil the pasta for 30 minutes in an excess of water and rinse it to remove the released starch. Then, we chill it in water to stop the cooking process and keep the noodles moist and soft. After cooling, the pasta is ready to be processed and re-heated.

SOFT & BITE-SIZED

LEVEL 6 – SOFT & BITE-SIZED

Description/characteristics
- Can be eaten with a fork, spoon or chopsticks
- Can be mashed/broken down with pressure from fork, spoon or chopsticks
- A knife is not required to cut this food, but may be used to help load a fork or spoon
- Soft, tender and moist throughout but with no separated thin liquid
- Chewing is required before swallowing
- 'Bite-sized' pieces as appropriate for size and oral processing skills
    - o Pediatric: 8 mm x 8 mm (no larger than)
    - o Adults: 15 mm x 15 mm (no larger than)

Physiological rationale for this level of thickness
- Biting is not required
- Chewing is required
- Food piece sizes designed to minimize choking risk
- Tongue force and control is required to move the food and keep it within the mouth for chewing and oral processing
- Tongue force is required to move the bolus for swallowing
- Pain or fatigue on chewing
- Missing teeth or poorly fitting dentures

Although descriptions are provided, use IDDSI Testing methods to decide if the food meets IDDSI
▼6 *Soft & Bite-Sized guidelines for adults.*

NOTES AND TIPS ON ▼6 SOFT & BITE-SIZED

Under IDDSI, someone on a ▼6 Soft & Bite-Sized diet can also eat any of the ▼5 Minced & Moist or ▼4 Pureed recipes. See pages 158–159 for more details.

THE RECIPES

Ground Beef

Meatloaf

Meatballs

Breaded Fish or Fish Sticks

Sauteed Fish

Scrambled Eggs

Egg Salad

Potato Salad

Chicken Salad

Tuna Salad

Carrots

Cauliflower

Broccoli

Green Beans

Butternut Squash

Peas

Snow or Sugar Snap Peas

Peaches

Pears

Lasagna

Buttered Noodles

Homemade Shells & Cheese

NOTES AND TIPS ON ⑥ SOFT & BITE-SIZED

The IDDSI requirements for ⑥ Soft & Bite-Sized are fairly straight-forward and easy to understand. The thinking behind this level is that although biting is not required, chewing is required to process the food. And the food should be soft enough to process very easily by chewing, without the patient becoming tired. Before getting into the notes and tips on this level, let's review exactly what qualifies for ⑥ Soft & Bite-Sized.

Here is a description from the 2019 IDDSI Consumer handout:

- Soft, tender and moist, but with no water-thin liquid leaking/dripping from the food
- Ability to 'bite off' a piece of food is not required
- Ability to chew 'bite-sized' pieces so that they are safe to swallow is required
- 'Bite-sized' pieces no bigger than 15 mm x 15 mm in size
- Food can be mashed/broken down with pressure from a fork
- A knife is not required to cut this food

The testing requirements for this level are:

1. No separated water-thin liquids.
2. All pieces must be smaller than 15 mm x 15 mm. This is the width of a typical dinner fork.
3. The food can be squashed and will not return to original shape when tested with a dinner fork or teaspoon with just enough pressure that the thumb nail turns white.
4. Food can be separated into smaller pieces using pressure from a dinner fork or a teaspoon held on its side.
5. Must meet all criteria for 30 minutes.

With these requirements in mind, there are many everyday foods that are very simple to process into ⑥ Soft & Bite-Sized by simply cutting them into small enough pieces. However, the thing that most often causes issues with ⑥ Soft & Bite-Sized is the "soft" part. The squashing and cutting requirements can make the preparation of some foods a little challenging.

MEATS

- Meats need to be cooked tender. This can be accomplished, but you will have to be careful to not overcook and make the meat too tough to pass the pressure and cutting tests. Typically, the easiest way to ensure tender meat, is to boil it in a vacuum-sealed bag (sous vide) or to use a juicy, slow-cooker recipe.

- But some meats and even some cuts of meat, simply won't ever be able to pass the squash test or be cut with gentle pressure on the side of a fork. Overcooked pork chops or a tough flank steak are examples of meats that are simply too tough for these requirements. Also, a grilled chicken breast may be cooked to slightly crispy on the edges to get the center completely cooked. If you have a meat that fails these tests, you can simply process it to ⑤ Minced & Moist. The meat will still taste great and will be very acceptable to the ⑥ Soft & Bite-Sized diet.

- In general, the suggestion is that you try to cook the meat very tender for your loved one. Then, test it and if it fails the squash test or the separation test, quickly process it to ⑤ Minced & Moist.

FRUIT

- Often fruit will be fine to simply cut and serve. But it is important to consider a person's individual needs.

- If fruit is too firm, serve minced or mashed. If you see water-thin liquids separating from the mash, mix with some △ Extremely Thick fruit juice or △ Extremely Thick Stock (see recipe on page 55) to absorb the water-thin fluids.

- Avoid fibrous fruit (like pineapple).

- Drain excess water-thin liquids.

- If you have fruit that is weeping water-thin liquids, put the pieces in a bowl and mix with some △ Extremely Thick fruit juice or △ Extremely Thick Stock (see recipe on page 55) to absorb the water-thin fluids.

VEGETABLES

- Cut to size, then steam or boil to "fork tender."

- If you have a vegetable that is weeping water-thin liquids, put the pieces in a bowl and mix with some ▽ Extremely Thick Stock (see recipe on page 55) to absorb the water-thin fluids.

PASTA DISHES

- Cut to size, drain water-thin liquids, be sure the other ingredients in the dish—meat, fish and vegetables—are tender and small enough to meet the ½" x ½" (15 mm x 15 mm) size requirements.

COLD BREAKFAST CEREALS

- Cereals should be soaked in milk for 10 minutes to soften the pieces. Milk needs to be drained, or with clinician approval can be thickened and served together.

RICE, OATMEAL, GRITS AND SIMILAR

- Cooked to very soft, with enough moisture to prevent stickiness, but drained of excess water-thin liquids.

BREADS & DESSERTS

- NO regular dry bread, sandwiches or toast of any kind! This includes cookies, brownies and cakes. Dry bread is too much of a choking risk.

- For sandwiches, use ▽ Pureed Bread (see recipe on page 60) with fillings that meet ▽ Soft & Bite-Sized or ▽ Minced & Moist requirements.

- It is possible to soak breads and cookies with milk to make them soft and not sticky.

SOFT & BITE-SIZED

Ground Beef

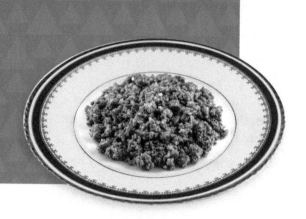

INGREDIENTS

- 16 oz. cooked ground beef, drained of grease (hot or cold meat can be used — bones and gristle must be removed)

NOTES

To meet ▼6 Soft & Bite-Sized requirements, ground beef needs to be cooked to a very tender texture. The challenge is to have cooked meat that will be easy to squash and separate with a fork. Many cooking techniques will result in meat that is too firm. Using very low heat may make this possible.

If you find during testing that the meat is too firm or too difficult to separate into smaller pieces, process the ground beef to ▼5 Minced & Moist. You can find the process for that on page 121.

Rely on the process and your test results to ensure proper preparation.

You can follow this process with ground meat substitutes as well.

DIRECTIONS

1. Place cooked ground beef onto cutting board.
2. Use knife to cut the ground beef into pieces no larger than 15 mm x 15 mm in size.
3. If some water-thin liquids are weeping and are present, drain and discard.
4. Evaluate to ensure compliance with IDDSI ▼6 Soft & Bite-Sized requirements:
   a. No separated water-thin liquids.
   b. All pieces are smaller than 15 mm x 15 mm.
   c. The pieces are easily squashed and will not return to original shape. Test by pushing down on a piece with a fork or teaspoon with enough pressure that the thumbnail turns white.
   d. Food can be separated into smaller pieces using pressure from a dinner fork or a teaspoon held on its side.
   e. Must meet all criteria for 30 minutes.
5. If the ground beef is too firm or difficult to separate, process the meat to ▼5 Minced & Moist. See page 121.
6. Serve, or store unused portions in refrigerator.

Meatloaf

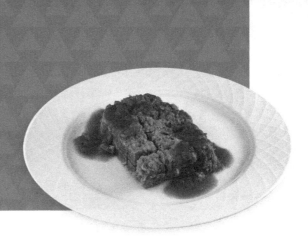

INGREDIENTS

- 13.2 oz. Stouffer's® meatloaf or equivalent — microwaved per instructions or fresh made from scratch meatloaf
- Depending on end use, 4 oz. Extremely Thick Sauce or Stock— see Basic Sauce recipe on page 51 for ketchup glaze or BBQ sauce, or Extremely Thick Stock recipe on page 55

NOTES

Meatloaf seems to be made for the Soft & Bite-Sized diet! Whether fresh, made from scratch or frozen, the soft texture is very well suited for this IDDSI level. The process for preparing frozen meatloaf to IDDSI Soft & Bite-Sized guidelines for adults involves simply draining any water-thin liquids and cutting the meatloaf to properly sized pieces. Rely on the process and your test results to ensure proper preparation.

DIRECTIONS

1. Place a serving of meatloaf onto a cutting board or dinner plate.
2. Use a knife or fork to cut meatloaf into pieces no larger than 15 mm x 15 mm in size.
3. Drain any water-thin liquids that are present.
4. Evaluate to ensure compliance with IDDSI Soft & Bite-Sized requirements:
   a. No separated water-thin liquids.
   b. All pieces are smaller than 15 mm x 15 mm.
   c. The pieces are easily squashed and will not return to original shape. Test by pushing down on a piece with a fork or teaspoon with enough pressure that the thumbnail turns white.
   d. Food can be separated into smaller pieces using pressure from a dinner fork or a teaspoon held on its side.
   e. Must meet all criteria for 30 minutes.
5. Top with ketchup glaze or BBQ sauce as desired.
6. Serve, or store unused portions in refrigerator.

Meatballs

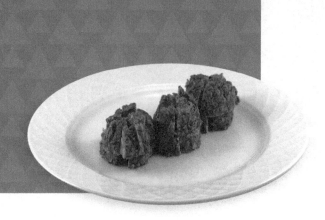

INGREDIENTS

- 12–16 oz. frozen or fresh made from scratch meatballs—cooked per package instructions
- Depending on end use, 4 oz. ④ Extremely Thick Sauce or Stock— see Marinara Sauce recipe on page 54, or ④ Extremely Thick Stock recipe on page 55

NOTES

Meatballs are a perfect meat for the ⑥ Soft & Bite-Sized diet! Whether fresh, made from scratch or frozen, the soft texture is very well suited for this IDDSI level. Meatballs can be used as a component of a pasta dish, a topping for ④ Pureed bread or simply covered with an appropriately thickened sauce. There are a variety of frozen meatballs available and each may behave a little differently, however this recipe is designed to be flexible and allow you to ensure compliance with IDDSI guidelines. Rely on the process and your test results to ensure proper preparation.

DIRECTIONS

1. Drain any thin sauce or drippings and place meatballs onto a cutting board.
2. Use a knife or fork to cut meatballs into pieces no larger than 15 mm x 15 mm in size.
3. Drain any water-thin liquids that are present.
4. Evaluate to ensure compliance with IDDSI ⑥ Soft & Bite-Sized requirements:
   a. No separated water-thin liquids.
   b. All pieces are smaller than 15 mm x 15 mm.
   c. The pieces are easily squashed and will not return to original shape. Test by pushing down on a piece with a fork or teaspoon with enough pressure that the thumbnail turns white.
   d. Food can be separated into smaller pieces using pressure from a dinner fork or a teaspoon held on its side.
   e. Must meet all criteria for 30 minutes.
5. Add to pasta or bread and top with ④ Extremely Thick Sauce (ketchup glaze, BBQ sauce or marinara) or ④ Extremely Thick Stock, as desired.
6. Serve, or store unused portions in refrigerator.

Breaded Fish or Fish Sticks

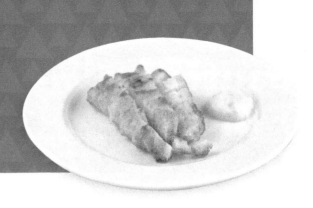

INGREDIENTS

- 16 oz. cooked frozen "beer battered" cod fillets, breaded fish sticks or equivalent—cooked according to the manufacturer's instructions

NOTES

Cooked fish, even with breading, tends to be very soft and moist. It is a great protein for the IDDSI ▼ Soft & Bite-Sized guidelines for adults. The major concern is whether any water-thin liquids are released by the fish. Rely on the process and your test results to ensure proper preparation.

DIRECTIONS

1. Place cooked fish onto cutting board.
2. Use knife to cut fish into pieces no larger than 15 mm x 15 mm in size.
3. Drain any water-thin liquids that are present.
4. Evaluate to ensure compliance with IDDSI ▼ Soft & Bite-Sized requirements:
   a. No separated water-thin liquids.
   b. All pieces are smaller than 15 mm x 15 mm.
   c. The pieces are easily squashed and will not return to original shape. Test by pushing down on a piece with a fork or teaspoon with enough pressure that the thumbnail turns white.
   d. Food can be separated into smaller pieces using pressure from a dinner fork or a teaspoon held on its side.
   e. Must meet all criteria for 30 minutes.
5. Serve, or store unused portions in refrigerator.

Sauteed Fish

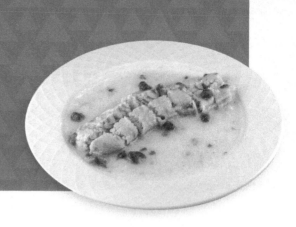

INGREDIENTS

- 16 oz. fish fillets, sauteed and "fork tender," drained of water-thin liquids (skin and bones must be removed)
- If necessary, △4 Extremely Thick Stock—see recipe on page 55

NOTES

Cooked fish tends to be very soft and moist. It is a great protein for the IDDSI ▽6 Soft & Bite-Sized guidelines for adults. The major concern is whether any water-thin liquids are released by the fish. If water-thin liquids keep seeping, a small amount of △4 Extremely Thick Stock can be used to control them. Rely on the process and your test results to ensure proper preparation.

DIRECTIONS

1. Place cooked fish onto cutting board.
2. Use knife to cut fish into pieces no larger than 15 mm x 15 mm in size.
3. Drain any water-thin liquids that are present.
4. Evaluate to ensure compliance with IDDSI ▽6 Soft & Bite-Sized requirements:
   a. No separated water-thin liquids.
   b. All pieces are smaller than 15 mm x 15 mm.
   c. The pieces are easily squashed and will not return to original shape. Test by pushing down on a piece with a fork or teaspoon with enough pressure that the thumbnail turns white.
   d. Food can be separated into smaller pieces using pressure from a dinner fork or a teaspoon held on its side.
   e. Must meet all criteria for 30 minutes.
5. If water-thin liquids continue to weep, transfer fish to a mixing bowl, add a small amount of △4 Extremely Thick Stock and mix carefully to avoid breaking down fish pieces further. Return to Step 4.
6. Serve, or store unused portions in refrigerator.

Scrambled Eggs

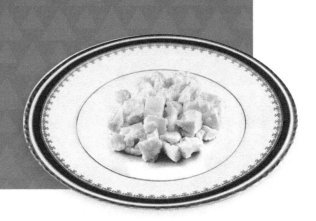

INGREDIENTS

- 4 eggs, scrambled and cooked (hot or cold)
- If necessary, 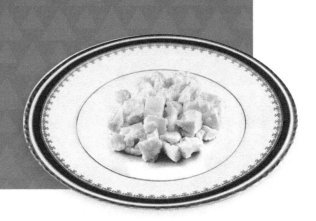 Extremely Thick Stock—see recipe on page 55

NOTES

Scrambled eggs are a natural Soft & Bite-Sized food. The only real concern is whether the eggs are cooked to the point that they weep water-thin liquids. If eggs weep water-thin liquids, some Extremely Thick Stock will need to be added to control the water-thin liquid. Rely on the process and your test results to ensure proper preparation.

Unused portions can be frozen and re-heated to serve. Typically, you will not need to add more liquid to scrambled eggs to meet IDDSI standards. However, it is common for scrambled eggs to "give up" water-thin liquids. Be prepared to drain water-thin liquids and monitor closely while eating to avoid choking risk.

DIRECTIONS

1. Add scrambled eggs to a bowl and observe for overly large egg pieces and the presence of water-thin liquids.
2. Use spatula or knife to break large pieces into pieces no larger than 15 mm x 15 mm in size.
3. If some water-thin liquids are weeping and are present, add small amounts of Extremely Thick Stock and combine with a spatula.
4. Evaluate to ensure compliance with IDDSI Soft & Bite-Sized requirements:
   a. No separated water-thin liquids.
   b. All pieces are smaller than 15 mm x 15 mm.
   c. The pieces are easily squashed and will not return to original shape. Test by pushing down on a piece with a fork or teaspoon with enough pressure that the thumbnail turns white.
   d. Food can be separated into smaller pieces using pressure from a dinner fork or a teaspoon held on its side.
   e. Must meet all criteria for 30 minutes.
5. Serve, or store unused portions in refrigerator.

SOFT & BITE-SIZED

Egg Salad

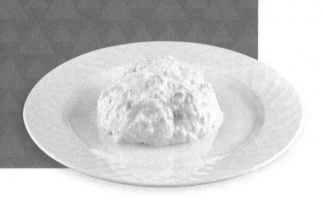

INGREDIENTS

• 16 oz. egg salad, homemade or store-bought

NOTES

Egg salad is a natural for the ▽6 Soft & Bite-Sized diet! Whether fresh homemade or store-bought, the soft texture is very well suited for this IDDSI level. The process for preparing egg salad to IDDSI ▽6 Soft & Bite-Sized guidelines for adults involves simply making sure all the pieces in the egg salad are properly cut to size. Rely on the process and your test results to ensure proper preparation.

DIRECTIONS

1. Place egg salad onto a cutting board or dinner plate.
2. Use a knife or fork to cut egg salad into pieces no larger than 15 mm x 15 mm in size.
3. Drain away any water-thin liquids that are present.
4. Evaluate to ensure compliance with IDDSI ▽6 Soft & Bite-Sized requirements:
   a. No separated water-thin liquids.
   b. All pieces are smaller than 15 mm x 15 mm.
   c. The pieces are easily squashed and will not return to original shape. Test by pushing down on a piece with a fork or teaspoon with enough pressure that the thumbnail turns white.
   d. Food can be separated into smaller pieces using pressure from a dinner fork or a teaspoon held on its side.
   e. Must meet all criteria for 30 minutes.
5. Serve, or store unused portions in refrigerator.

Potato Salad

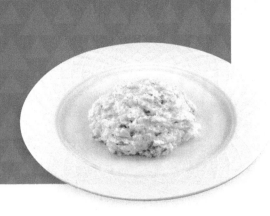

INGREDIENTS

- 16 oz. potato salad, homemade or store-bought

NOTES

Potato salad is a natural for the ⑥ Soft & Bite-Sized diet! However, we must be on the lookout for over-sized and undercooked potato pieces. Whether fresh homemade or store-bought, when fully cooked, the soft texture is very well suited for this IDDSI level. The process for preparing potato salad to IDDSI ⑥ Soft & Bite-Sized guidelines for adults involves simply making sure all the pieces in the potato salad are properly cut to size and the potato pieces are fully cooked. Rely on the process and your test results to ensure proper preparation.

DIRECTIONS

1. Place potato salad onto a cutting board or dinner plate.
2. Use a knife or fork to cut potato salad into pieces no larger than 15 mm x 15 mm in size.
3. Set aside any firmer potato pieces for evaluation in Step 5.
4. Drain away any water-thin liquids that are present.
5. Evaluate to ensure compliance with IDDSI ⑥ Soft & Bite-Sized requirements:
   a. No separated water-thin liquids.
   b. All pieces are smaller than 15 mm x 15 mm.
   c. The pieces are easily squashed and will not return to original shape. Test by pushing down on a piece with a fork or teaspoon with enough pressure that the thumbnail turns white.
   d. Food can be separated into smaller pieces using pressure from a dinner fork or a teaspoon held on its side.
   e. Must meet all criteria for 30 minutes.
6. Serve, or store unused portions in refrigerator.

Chicken Salad

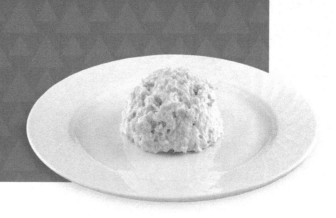

INGREDIENTS

- 16 oz. chicken salad, homemade or store-bought.

NOTES

Chicken salad is a natural for the ▼ 6 Soft & Bite-Sized diet! Whether fresh homemade or store-bought, the soft texture is very well suited for this IDDSI level. However, chicken salad is often commercially prepared with raw peppers, celery and nuts. All of these individual pieces will fail the requirements to be easily squashed and cut by a fork. It is best to purchase or make chicken salad without these ingredients. However, they can be removed easily during preparation. Rely on the process and your test results to ensure proper preparation.

DIRECTIONS

1. Place chicken salad onto a cutting board or dinner plate.
2. Use a knife or fork to cut chicken salad into pieces no larger than 15 mm x 15 mm in size.
3. Remove any obviously tough or firm ingredients like raw peppers, celery and/or nuts.
4. Drain away any water-thin liquids that are present.
5. Evaluate to ensure compliance with IDDSI 6 ▼ Soft & Bite-Sized requirements:
   a. No separated water-thin liquids.
   b. All pieces are smaller than 15 mm x 15 mm.
   c. The pieces are easily squashed and will not return to original shape. Test by pushing down on a piece with a fork or teaspoon with enough pressure that the thumbnail turns white.
   d. Food can be separated into smaller pieces using pressure from a dinner fork or a teaspoon held on its side.
   e. Must meet all criteria for 30 minutes.
6. Serve, or store unused portions in refrigerator.

Tuna Salad

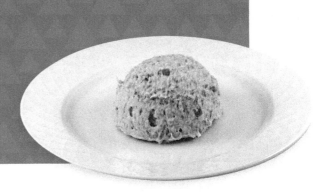

INGREDIENTS

- 16 oz. tuna salad, homemade or store-bought

NOTES

Tuna salad is a natural for the ▽6 Soft & Bite-Sized diet! Whether fresh homemade or store-bought, the soft texture is very well suited for this IDDSI level. Tuna salad is often commercially prepared with raw peppers, celery and nuts. All of these individual pieces will fail the requirements to be easily squashed and cut by a fork. It is best to purchase or make tuna salad without these ingredients. However, they can be removed easily during preparation. Rely on the process and your test results to ensure proper preparation.

DIRECTIONS

1. Place tuna salad onto a cutting board or dinner plate.
2. Use a knife or fork to cut tuna salad into pieces no larger than 15 mm x 15 mm in size.
3. Remove any obviously tough or firm ingredients like raw peppers, celery and/or nuts.
4. Drain away any water-thin liquids that are present.
5. Evaluate to ensure compliance with IDDSI ▽6 Soft & Bite-Sized requirements:
   a. No separated water-thin liquids.
   b. All pieces are smaller than 15 mm x 15 mm.
   c. The pieces are easily squashed and will not return to original shape. Test by pushing down on a piece with a fork or teaspoon with enough pressure that the thumbnail turns white.
   d. Food can be separated into smaller pieces using pressure from a dinner fork or a teaspoon held on its side.
   e. Must meet all criteria for 30 minutes.
6. Serve, or store unused portions in refrigerator.

Carrots

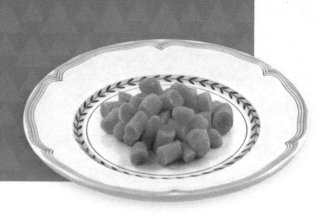

INGREDIENTS

- 2 cups (16 oz.) carrots, cooked until tender enough to be pierced or cut easily with a fork (hot or cold)
- Extremely Thick Stock— see recipe on page 55

NOTES

The process for cooked carrots to meet IDDSI ⑥ Soft & Bite-Sized guidelines is mostly knife-cutting to ensure proper sized pieces. Most of the time, cooked carrots will not weep any water-thin liquid. However, it does happen on some occasions. When this happens, some ④ Extremely Thick Stock will need to be added to control the water-thin liquid. This process will work with both hot or cold carrots. Rely on the process and your test results to ensure proper preparation.

DIRECTIONS

1. Add carrots to a colander, rinse and drain thoroughly.
2. Use knife to cut cooked carrots into pieces no larger than 15 mm x 15 mm in size.
3. If water-thin liquids are weeping and present:
   a. Put cut carrots in a bowl.
   b. Add small amounts of ④ Extremely Thick Stock and combine with a spatula.
4. Evaluate to ensure compliance with IDDSI ⑥ Soft & Bite-Sized requirements:
   a. No separated water-thin liquids.
   b. All pieces are smaller than 15 mm x 15 mm.
   c. The pieces are easily squashed and will not return to original shape. Test by pushing down on a piece with a fork or teaspoon with enough pressure that the thumbnail turns white.
   d. Food can be separated into smaller pieces using pressure from a dinner fork or a teaspoon held on its side.
   e. Must meet all criteria for 30 minutes.
5. Serve, or store unused portions in refrigerator.

Cauliflower

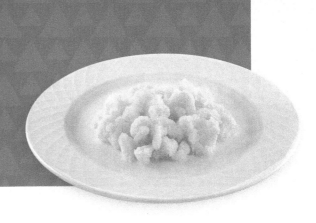

INGREDIENTS

- 2 cups (16 oz.) cauliflower, cooked until tender enough to be pierced or cut easily with a fork (hot or cold)
- If necessary, Extremely Thick Stock—see recipe on page 55

NOTES

The process for cooked cauliflower to meet IDDSI 6 Soft & Bite-Sized guidelines is mostly a knife-cutting process to ensure proper sized pieces. Depending on the source of the cauliflower and the cooking method, some cauliflower will weep water-thin liquid. When this happens, some Extremely Thick Stock will need to be added to control the water-thin liquid. This process will work with both hot or cold cauliflower. Rely on the process and your test results to ensure proper preparation.

DIRECTIONS

1. Add cooked cauliflower to a colander, rinse and drain thoroughly.
2. Use knife to cut cooked cauliflower into pieces no larger than 15 mm x 15 mm in size.
3. If water-thin liquids are weeping and present:
   a. Put cut cauliflower in a bowl.
   b. Add small amounts of Extremely Thick Stock and combine with a spatula.
4. Evaluate to ensure compliance with IDDSI 6 Soft & Bite-Sized requirements:
   a. No separated water-thin liquids.
   b. All pieces are smaller than 15 mm x 15 mm.
   c. The pieces are easily squashed and will not return to original shape. Test by pushing down on a piece with a fork or teaspoon with enough pressure that the thumbnail turns white.
   d. Food can be separated into smaller pieces using pressure from a dinner fork or a teaspoon held on its side.
   e. Must meet all criteria for 30 minutes.
5. Serve, or store unused portions in refrigerator.

Broccoli

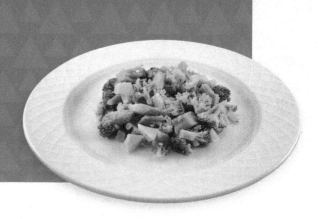

INGREDIENTS

- 2 cups (16 oz.) broccoli, cooked until the thicker stems are tender enough to be pierced or cut easily with a fork (hot or cold)
- If necessary, 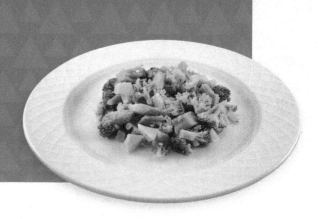 Extremely Thick Stock—see recipe on page 55

NOTES

The process for cooked broccoli to meet IDDSI 6 Soft & Bite-Sized guidelines is mostly knife-cutting to ensure proper sized pieces. Depending on the source of the broccoli (fresh or frozen) and the cooking method, some broccoli will weep water-thin liquid. When this happens, some Extremely Thick Stock will need to be added to control the water-thin liquid. This process will work with both hot or cold cooked broccoli. Rely on the process and your test results to ensure proper preparation.

DIRECTIONS

1. Add cooked broccoli to a colander, rinse and drain thoroughly.
2. Use knife to cut cooked broccoli into pieces no larger than 15 mm x 15 mm in size.
3. If water-thin liquids are weeping and present:
   a. Put cut broccoli in a bowl.
   b. Add small amounts of Extremely Thick Stock and combine with a spatula.
4. Evaluate to ensure compliance with IDDSI 6 Soft & Bite-Sized requirements:
   a. No separated water-thin liquids.
   b. All pieces are smaller than 15 mm x 15 mm.
   c. The pieces are easily squashed and will not return to original shape. Test by pushing down on a piece with a fork or teaspoon with enough pressure that the thumbnail turns white.
   d. Food can be separated into smaller pieces using pressure from a dinner fork or a teaspoon held on its side.
   e. Must meet all criteria for 30 minutes.
5. Serve, or store unused portions in refrigerator.

Green Beans

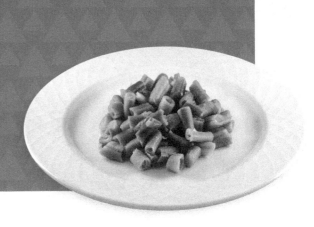

INGREDIENTS

- 2 cups (16 oz.) green beans, cooked until tender enough to be pierced or cut easily with a fork, drained of all drippings and thin liquids (hot or cold)
- If necessary, ④ Extremely Thick Stock—see recipe on page 55

NOTES

The process for cooked green beans to meet IDDSI ⑥ Soft & Bite-Sized guidelines is mostly knife-cutting to ensure proper sized pieces. Depending on the source of the green beans (canned, fresh or frozen) and the cooking method, some green beans will weep water-thin liquid. When this happens, some ④ Extremely Thick Stock will need to be added to control the water-thin liquid. This process will work with both hot or cold green beans. Rely on the process and your test results to ensure proper preparation.

DIRECTIONS

1. Add cooked green beans to a colander, rinse and drain thoroughly.
2. Use knife to cut cooked green beans into pieces no larger than 15 mm x 15 mm in size.
3. If water-thin liquids are weeping and present:
   a. Put cut green beans in a bowl.
   b. Add small amounts of ④ Extremely Thick Stock and combine with a spatula.
4. Evaluate to ensure compliance with IDDSI ⑥ Soft & Bite-Sized requirements:
   a. No separated water-thin liquids.
   b. All pieces are smaller than 15 mm x 15 mm.
   c. The pieces are easily squashed and will not return to original shape. Test by pushing down on a piece with a fork or teaspoon with enough pressure that the thumbnail turns white.
   d. Food can be separated into smaller pieces using pressure from a dinner fork or a teaspoon held on its side.
   e. Must meet all criteria for 30 minutes.
5. Serve, or store unused portions in refrigerator.

Butternut Squash

INGREDIENTS

- 2 cups (16 oz.) butternut squash, cooked until tender enough to be cut easily with a fork and drained thoroughly (hot or cold)

NOTES

This process will work with both hot or cold butternut squash. Preference is given for steamed or microwave preparation. Testing with frozen and/or oven-baked butternut squash often resulted in crusty corners and edges with a drier final product. Because of these results, we do not recommend using an oven-baked butternut squash for ▽6 Soft & Bite-Sized butternut squash. Rely on the process and your test results to ensure proper preparation.

DIRECTIONS

1. Use dinner knife and fork to cut cooked butternut squash into pieces no larger than 15 mm x 15 mm.
2. When all pieces are the correct size, drain all water-thin liquids released from the cooked butternut squash as they are not allowed by ▽6 Soft & Bite-Sized.
3. Evaluate to ensure compliance with IDDSI ▽6 Soft & Bite-Sized requirements:
   a. No separated water-thin liquids.
   b. All pieces are smaller than 15 mm x 15 mm.
   c. The pieces are easily squashed and will not return to original shape. Test by pushing down on a piece with a fork or teaspoon with enough pressure that the thumbnail turns white.
   d. Food can be separated into smaller pieces using pressure from a dinner fork or a teaspoon held on its side.
   e. Must meet all criteria for 30 minutes.
4. Serve, or store unused portions in refrigerator.

Bonus presentation tip: Sprinkle with cinnamon (if approved by your SLP).

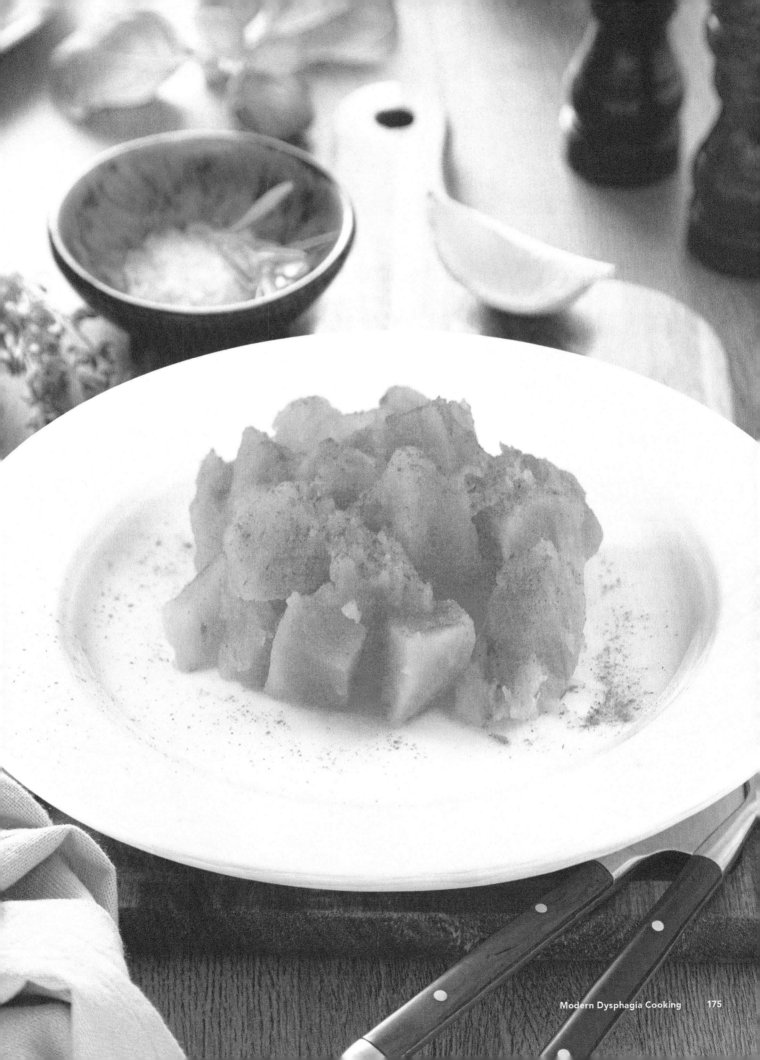

Peas

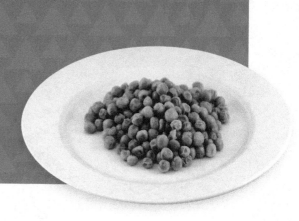

INGREDIENTS

- 2 cups (16 oz.) peas, cooked until tender enough to be pierced or cut easily with a fork and drained thoroughly (hot or cold)
- If necessary, ▲4 Extremely Thick Stock—see recipe on page 55

NOTES

The process for peas is to meet IDDSI ▼6 Soft & Bite-Sized is simply quality control. Peas are almost always small enough to meet IDDSI requirements without further cutting. Very rarely, some peas will weep water-thin liquid. Fresh, frozen or canned peas can be used. Each will require a slightly different amount of washing and draining to remove water-thin liquids. When this happens, some ▲4 Extremely Thick Stock will need to be added to control the water-thin liquid. This process will work with both hot or cold peas. Rely on the process and your test results to ensure proper preparation.

DIRECTIONS

1. Add cooked peas to a colander, rinse and drain thoroughly.
2. Inspect for over-sized peas that are greater than 15 mm x 15 mm in size. If any are found, cut with a knife.
3. Very rarely, some water-thin liquids may continue to weep. If this is the case:
   a. Put peas in a bowl.
   b. Add small amounts of ▲4 Extremely Thick Stock and combine with a spatula.
4. Evaluate to ensure compliance with IDDSI ▼6 Soft & Bite-Sized requirements:
   a. No separated water-thin liquids.
   b. All pieces are smaller than 15 mm x 15 mm.
   c. The pieces are easily squashed and will not return to original shape. Test by pushing down on a piece with a fork or teaspoon with enough pressure that the thumbnail turns white.
   d. Food can be separated into smaller pieces using pressure from a dinner fork or a teaspoon held on its side.
   e. Must meet all criteria for 30 minutes.
5. Serve, or store unused portions in refrigerator.

Snow or Sugar Snap Peas

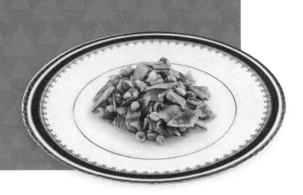

INGREDIENTS

- 2 cups (16 oz.) snow or sugar snap peas, cooked in the pod until tender enough to be pierced or cut easily with a fork and drained thoroughly (hot or cold)
- If necessary, 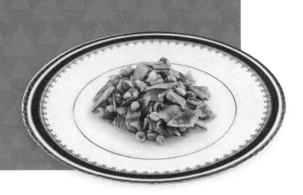 Extremely Thick Stock—see recipe on page 55

NOTES

The process for snow or sugar snap peas to meet IDDSI Soft & Bite-Sized guidelines is simply quality control. Snow and sugar snap peas are cooked in the pod and will need to be cut to meet IDDSI size requirements. Very rarely, some snow or sugar snap peas will weep water-thin liquid. When this happens, some Extremely Thick Stock will need to be added to control the water-thin liquid. This process will work with both hot or cold peas. Rely on the process and your test results to ensure proper preparation.

DIRECTIONS

1. Add cooked snow or sugar snap peas to a colander, rinse and drain thoroughly.
2. Use knife to cut cooked snow or sugar snap peas into pieces no larger than 15 mm x 15 mm in size.
3. Inspect for over-sized peas that are greater than 15 mm x 15 mm in size. If any are found, cut with a knife.
4. Very rarely, some water-thin liquids may continue to weep. If this is the case:
   a. Put snow or sugar snap peas in a bowl.
   b. Add small amounts of Extremely Thick Stock and combine with a spatula.
5. Evaluate to ensure compliance with IDDSI Soft & Bite-Sized requirements:
   a. No separated water-thin liquids.
   b. All pieces are smaller than 15 mm x 15 mm.
   c. The pieces are easily squashed and will not return to original shape. Test by pushing down on a piece with a fork or teaspoon with enough pressure that the thumbnail turns white.
   d. Food can be separated into smaller pieces using pressure from a dinner fork or a teaspoon held on its side.
   e. Must meet all criteria for 30 minutes.
6. Serve, or store unused portions in refrigerator.

Peaches

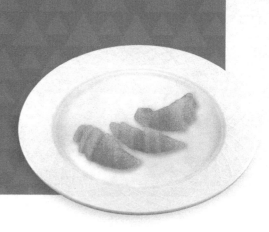

INGREDIENTS

- 2 cups (16 oz.) of peaches—thawed, peeled, rinsed and drained, as appropriate
- ⚠️ Extremely Thick Stock—see recipe on page 55

NOTES

IDDSI ▼6 Soft & Bite-Sized guidelines require a knife-cutting process to ensure proper sized pieces. Depending on the source of the peaches, some peaches may weep water-thin liquid. When this happens, some ⚠️ Extremely Thick Stock will need to be added to control the water-thin liquid. Depending on the person and their ability to orally process food, consider peeling the skins off fresh peaches. Rely on the process and your test results to ensure proper preparation.

DIRECTIONS

1. Add peaches to a colander and rinse and drain thoroughly.
2. Use knife to cut peaches into pieces no larger than 15 mm x 15 mm in size.
3. If some water-thin liquids are weeping and are present:
   a. Put cut peaches in a bowl.
   b. Add small amounts of ⚠️ Extremely Thick Stock and combine with a spatula.
4. Evaluate to ensure compliance with IDDSI ▼6 Soft & Bite-Sized requirements:
   a. No separated water-thin liquids.
   b. All pieces are smaller than 15 mm x 15 mm.
   c. The pieces are easily squashed and will not return to original shape. Test by pushing down on a piece with a fork or teaspoon with enough pressure that the thumbnail turns white.
   d. Food can be separated into smaller pieces using pressure from a dinner fork or a teaspoon held on its side.
   e. Must meet all criteria for 30 minutes.
5. Serve, or store unused portions in refrigerator.

Pears

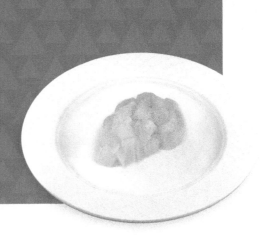

INGREDIENTS

- 2 cups (16 oz.) of pears—peeled and cored, rinsed and drained, as appropriate
- 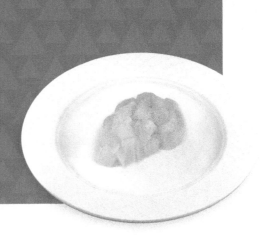 Extremely Thick Stock—see recipe on page 55

NOTES

IDDSI ▼ Soft & Bite-Sized guidelines require a knife-cutting process to ensure proper sized pieces. Depending on the source of the pears, some pears may weep water-thin liquid. When this happens, some ▲ Extremely Thick Stock will need to be added to control the water-thin liquid. Depending on the person and their ability to orally process foods, consider peeling the skins off fresh pears. Fresh pears require the removal of the pit and any stringy parts of the fruit. Rely on the process and your test results to ensure proper preparation.

DIRECTIONS

1. Add pears to a colander and rinse and drain thoroughly.
2. Use knife to cut pears into pieces no larger than 15 mm x 15 mm in size.
3. If some water-thin liquids are weeping and are present:
   a. Put cut pears in a bowl.
   b. Add small amounts of ▲ Extremely Thick Stock and combine with a spatula.
4. Evaluate to ensure compliance with IDDSI ▼ Soft & Bite-Sized requirements:
   a. No separated water-thin liquids.
   b. All pieces are smaller than 15 mm x 15 mm.
   c. The pieces are easily squashed and will not return to original shape. Test by pushing down on a piece with a fork or teaspoon with enough pressure that the thumbnail turns white.
   d. Food can be separated into smaller pieces using pressure from a dinner fork or a teaspoon held on its side.
   e. Must meet all criteria for 30 minutes.
5. Serve, or store unused portions in refrigerator.

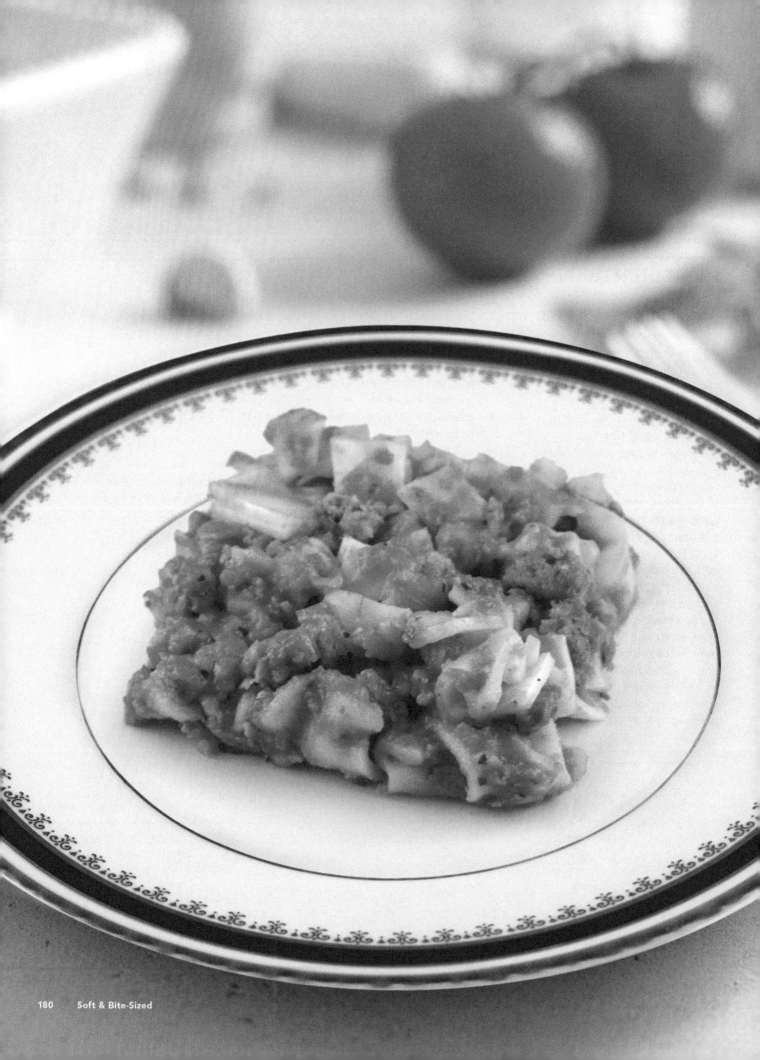

Lasagna

INGREDIENTS

- 1 lasagna (typically 24 oz.), homemade or store-bought —cooked per instructions

NOTES

Meeting ▽6 Soft & Bite-Sized standards involves cutting the lasagna to properly sized pieces. Some water-thin liquid is likely to separate from the lasagna. When this happens, simply drain away the water-thin liquid. Rely on the process and your test results to ensure proper preparation.

DIRECTIONS

1. Place a serving of lasagna onto a cutting board or dinner plate.
2. Use a knife or fork to cut lasagna into pieces no larger than 15 mm x 15 mm in size.
3. Drain away any water-thin liquids that are present.
4. Evaluate to ensure compliance with IDDSI ▽6 Soft & Bite-Sized requirements:
   a. No separated water-thin liquids.
   b. All pieces are smaller than 15 mm x 15 mm.
   c. The pieces are easily squashed and will not return to original shape. Test by pushing down on a piece with a fork or teaspoon with enough pressure that the thumbnail turns white.
   d. Food can be separated into smaller pieces using pressure from a dinner fork or a teaspoon held on its side.
   e. Must meet all criteria for 30 minutes.
5. Serve, or store unused portions in refrigerator.

Buttered Noodles

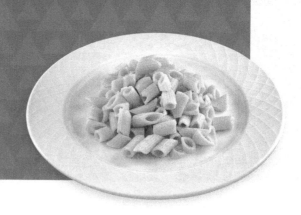

INGREDIENTS

- 4 oz. (approx. 1 cup) dry pasta (shapes, like elbow macaroni, farfalle, etc., are easiest to work with)
- 2–4 oz. milk
- 2 tablespoons butter
- Water

NOTES

Noodles are a natural dish to meet IDDSI 6 Soft & Bite-Sized guidelines. The two main concerns are the size of the noodle pieces and the potential for the noodles to become sticky before eating.

A little knife-work will reduce the noodle size and a little extra milk and/or butter will help reduce the stickiness. In addition, cooking with excess water and rinsing after cooking will help ensure every noodle is well cooked and most of the starch released during cooking is washed away. Rely on the process and your test results to ensure proper preparation.

DIRECTIONS

1. Prepare pasta with twice the recommend amount of water per package directions.
2. Drain pasta in colander.
3. Rinse pasta in colander thoroughly with cold water.
4. Place rinsed noodles onto a cutting board.
5. Use a knife or fork to cut noodles into pieces no larger than 15 mm x 15 mm in size.
6. Add noodles to microwave-safe mixing bowl.
7. Add butter and milk, 1 oz. at a time, and stir with a spatula until well-mixed and stickiness is reduced. If necessary, heat briefly in microwave to melt butter and warm noodles.
8. Evaluate to ensure compliance with IDDSI 6 Soft & Bite-Sized requirements:
   a. No separated water-thin liquids.
   b. All pieces are smaller than 15 mm x 15 mm.
   c. The pieces are easily squashed and will not return to original shape. Test by pushing down on a piece with a fork or teaspoon with enough pressure that the thumbnail turns white.
   d. Food can be separated into smaller pieces using pressure from a dinner fork or a teaspoon held on its side.
   e. Must meet all criteria for 30 minutes.
9. Serve, or store unused portions in refrigerator.

Homemade Shells & Cheese

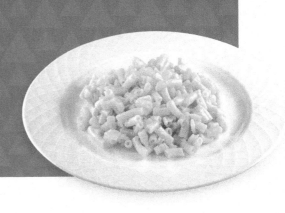

INGREDIENTS

- 2 cups macaroni & cheese, cooked or heated according to recipe or package instructions
- 2–4 oz. milk

NOTES

Shells & cheese is a natural dish to meet IDDSI **6** Soft & Bite-Sized guidelines. The two main concerns are the size of the noodle pieces and the potential for the dish to become sticky as it cools. A little knife-work will reduce the noodle size and a little extra milk will help reduce the stickiness. Rely on the process and your test results to ensure proper preparation.

DIRECTIONS

1. Place prepared shells & cheese onto a cutting board or dinner plate.
2. Use a knife or fork to cut cooked shell pasta noodles into pieces no larger than 15 mm x 15 mm in size.
3. Add milk, 1 oz. at a time, and stir with a spatula until well mixed and stickiness is reduced.
4. Evaluate to ensure compliance with IDDSI **6** Soft & Bite-Sized requirements:
   a. No separated water-thin liquids.
   b. All pieces are smaller than 15 mm x 15 mm.
   c. The pieces are easily squashed and will not return to original shape. Test by pushing down on a piece with a fork or teaspoon with enough pressure that the thumbnail turns white.
   d. Food can be separated into smaller pieces using pressure from a dinner fork or a teaspoon held on its side.
   e. Must meet all criteria for 30 minutes.
5. Serve, or store unused portions in refrigerator.

IDDSI Detailed Descriptors by Level

In this appendix, we have reprinted information for Pureed, Minced & Moist and Soft & Bite-Sized diet levels directly from the Complete IDDSI Framework Detail Definitions 2.0 | 2019.

Our intention here is a a faithful reproduction of the document found on www.iddsi.org. However, it has been reformatted to fit the style, format and size of our book. For the most current information, we always suggest you consult www.iddsi.org.

▼④ Pureed
▲④ Extremely Thick

Description/characteristics

- Usually eaten with a spoon (a fork is possible)
- Cannot be drunk from a cup, because it does not flow easily
- Cannot be sucked through a straw
- Does not require chewing
- Can be piped, layered or molded because it retains its shape, but should not require chewing if presented in this form
- Shows some very slow movement under gravity, but cannot be poured
- Falls off spoon in a single spoonful when tilted and continues to hold shape on a plate
- No lumps
- Not sticky
- Liquid must not separate from solid

Physiological rationale for this level of thickness

- If tongue control is significantly reduced, this category may be easiest to control
- Requires less propulsion effort than ▼⑤ Minced & Moist, ▼⑥ Soft & Bite-Sized, and ▼ Regular Easy to Chew, but more than ③ Liquidised/Moderately Thick
- No biting or chewing is required
- Increased oral and/or pharyngeal residue is a risk if too sticky
- Any food that requires chewing, controlled manipulation, or bolus formation are not suitable
- Pain on chewing or swallowing
- Missing teeth, or poorly fitting dentures

Although descriptions are provided, use IDDSI Testing methods to decide if the food meets IDDSI ▼④ Pureed guidelines.

▼ PUREED / ▲ EXTREMELY THICK TESTING METHODS

See also IDDSI Testing Methods document or
www.iddsi.org/framework/food-testing-methods/

IDDSI Flow Test

- The IDDSI Flow Test is NOT applicable, please use the Fork Drip Test and Spoon Tilt Test.

Fork Pressure Test

- Smooth with no lumps and minimal granulation.

- When a fork is pressed on the surface of Level 4 Extremely Thick Liquid/Pureed food, the tines/prongs of a fork can make a clear pattern on the surface, and/or the food retains the indentation from the fork.

Fork Drip Test

- Sample sits in a mound/pile above the fork; a small amount may flow through and form a short tail below the fork tines/prongs, but it **does not** flow or drip **continuously** through the prongs of a fork (see photo on page 187).

Spoon Tilt Test

- Cohesive enough to hold its shape on the spoon.

- A full spoonful must plop off the spoon if the spoon is tilted or turned sideways; a very gentle flick (using only fingers and wrist) may be necessary to dislodge the sample from the spoon, but the sample should slide off easily with very little food left on the spoon. A thin film remaining on the spoon after the Spoon Tilt Test is acceptable, however, you should still be able to see the spoon through the thin film; i.e. the sample should **not** be firm and sticky.

- May spread out slightly or slump very slowly on a flat plate.

Chopstick Test (where forks are not available)

- Chopsticks are not suitable for this texture.

Finger Test (where forks are not available)

- It is just possible to hold a sample of this texture using fingers. The texture slides smoothly and easily between the fingers and leaves a noticeable coating.

Indicators that a sample is too thick

- Does not fall off the spoon when tilted.

- Sticks to spoon.

FOOD SPECIFIC, OR OTHER EXAMPLES

The following item may be suitable for IDDSI ▼ Pureed:

- Purees suitable for infants (e.g. pureed meat, thick cereal)

FIGURES & DEMONSTRATIONS

- Sits in a mound or pile above the fork.

- A small amount may flow through and form a short tail below the fork. Does not dollop, flow or drip continuously through the fork prongs.

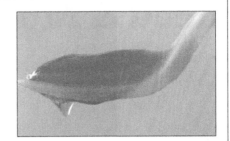

Spoon Tilt Test:

The following images show examples of foods that would be suitable or unsuitable for Level 4 according to the IDDSI Spoon Tilt Test.

SAFE: Holds shape on spoon; not firm and sticky; little food left on spoon.

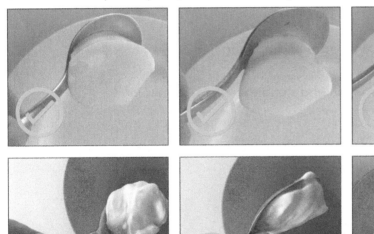

UNSAFE: Holds shape on spoon; FIRM AND STICKY; LOTS OF food left on spoon.

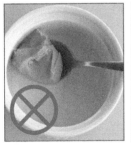 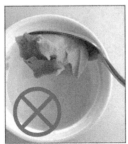 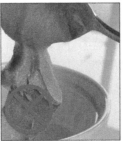 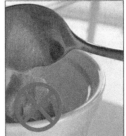

▽ Minced & Moist

Description/characteristics

- Can be eaten with a fork or spoon
- Could be eaten with chopsticks in some cases, if the individual has very good hand control
- Can be scooped and shaped (e.g. into a ball shape) on a plate
- Soft and moist with no separated water-thin liquid
- Small lumps visible within the food
  - **Pediatric: equal to or less than 2 mm width and no longer than 8 mm in length**
  - **Adult: equal to or less than 4 mm width and no longer than 15 mm in length**
- Lumps are easy to squash with tongue

Physiological rationale for this level of thickness

- Biting is not required
- Minimal chewing is required
- Tongue force alone can be used to separate the soft small particles in this texture
- Tongue force is required to move the bolus
- Pain or fatigue on chewing
- Missing teeth, or poorly fitting dentures

Although descriptions are provided, use IDDSI Testing methods to decide if the food meets IDDSI ▽ Minced & Moist guidelines.

▽ MINCED & MOIST TESTING METHODS

See also IDDSI Testing Methods document or
www.iddsi.org/framework/food-testing-methods/

Fork Pressure Test

- When pressed with a fork, the particles should easily separate between, and come through, the tines/prongs of a fork.

- Can be easily mashed with little pressure from a fork (pressure should **not** make the thumb nail blanch to white).

Fork Drip Test

- When a sample is scooped with a fork, it sits in a pile or can mound on the fork and does not easily or completely flow or fall through the tines/prongs of a fork.

Spoon Tilt Test

- Cohesive enough to hold its shape on the spoon.

- A full spoonful must slide/pour off/fall off the spoon if the spoon is tilted or turned sideways or shaken lightly; the sample should slide off easily with very little food left on the spoon; i.e. the sample should **not** be sticky.

- A scooped mound may spread or slump very slightly on a plate.

Chopstick Test (where forks are not available)

- Chopsticks can be used to scoop or hold this texture if the sample is moist and cohesive and the person has very good hand control to use chopsticks.

Finger Test (where forks are not available)

- It is possible to easily hold a sample of this texture using fingers; small, soft, smooth, rounded particles can be easily separated using fingers. The material will feel moist and leave fingers wet.

FOOD SPECIFIC, OR OTHER EXAMPLES

The following items may be suitable for IDDSI ▽ Minced & Moist:

Meat

- Finely minced*, chopped*, or soft mince
  - Pediatric: equal to or less than 2 mm width and no longer than 8 mm in length
  - Adult: equal to or less than 4 mm width and no more than 15 mm in length
- Serve in mildly, moderately or extremely thick, smooth, sauce or gravy, draining excess liquid

* If texture cannot be finely minced, it should be pureed.

Fish

- Finely mashed in mildly, moderately or extremely thick smooth, sauce or gravy, draining excess liquid
  - Pediatric: equal to or less than 2 mm width and no longer than 8 mm in length
  - Adult: equal to or less than 4 mm width and no more than 15 mm in length

Fruit

- Serve finely minced, chopped or mashed
- Drain excess juice
- If needed, serve in mildly, moderately or extremely thick smooth sauce or gravy AND drain excess liquid. No thin liquid should separate from food
  - Pediatric: equal to or less than 2 mm width and no longer than 8 mm in length
  - Adult: equal to or less than 4 mm width and no more than 15 mm in length

Vegetables

- Serve finely minced, chopped or mashed
- Drain any liquid
- If needed, serve in mildly, moderately or extremely thick smooth sauce or gravy AND drain excess liquid. No thin liquid should separate from food
  - Pediatric: equal to or less than 2 mm width and no longer than 8 mm in length
  - Adult: equal to or less than 4 mm width and no more than 15 mm in length

Cereal

- Thick and smooth with small soft lumps
  - Pediatric, equal to or less than 2 mm width and no longer than 8 mm in length
  - Adult, equal to or less than 4 mm width and no more than 15 mm in length
- Texture fully softened
- Any milk/liquid must not separate away from cereal. Drain any excess liquid before serving

Bread

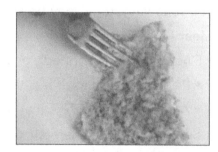

- No regular, dry bread, sandwiches or toast of any kind
- Use IDDSI ⑤ Minced & Moist sandwich recipe video (https://youtu.be/W7bOufqmz18)
- Pre-gelled 'soaked' breads that are very moist and gelled through the entire process

Rice, Couscous, Quinoa

- Not sticky or glutinous
- Should not be particulate or separate into individual grains when cooked and served
- Serve with smooth mildly, moderately or extremely thick sauce AND sauce must not separate away from couscous, quinoa (and similar food textures); drain excess liquid before serving

▼ MINCED & MOIST MEASUREMENT

Use slot between fork prongs (4 mm) to determine whether minced pieces are the correct or incorrect size

Note: Lump size requirements for all foods in Level 5 Minced & Moist:

- Pediatric: Equal to or less than 2 mm width and no more than 8 mm in length
- Adult: Equal to or less than 4 mm width and no more than 15 mm in length

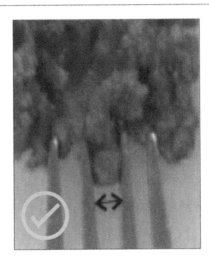 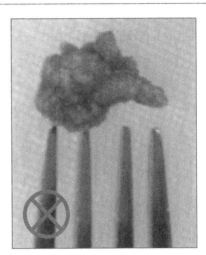

▼ MINCED & MOIST FOOD MUST PASS ALL THREE TESTS!

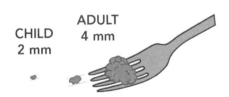

CHILD 2 mm — ADULT 4 mm

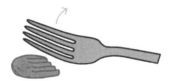

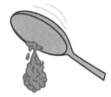

1. IDDSI Fork Test

- Pediatric: Equal to or less than 2 mm width and no more than 8 mm in length
- Adult: Equal to or less than 4 mm width and no more than 15 mm length

4 mm is about the gap between the prongs of a standard dinner fork

2. IDDSI Fork Test

- Soft enough to squash easily with fork or spoon

Don't need a thumb nail to blanch white

3. IDDSI Spoon Test

- Sample holds its shape on the spoon and falls off fairly easily if the spoon is tilted or lightly flicked
- Sample should not be firm or sticky

▼ 6 Soft & Bite-Sized

Description/characteristics

- Can be eaten with a fork, spoon or chopsticks
- Can be mashed/broken down with pressure from fork, spoon or chopsticks
- A knife is not required to cut this food, but may be used to help load a fork or spoon
- Soft, tender and moist throughout but with no separated thin liquid
- Chewing is required before swallowing
- 'Bite-sized' pieces as appropriate for size and oral processing skills
  - **Pediatric: 8 mm pieces (no larger than)**
  - **Adults: 15 mm = 1.5 cm pieces (no larger than)**

Physiological rationale for this level of thickness

- Biting is not required
- Chewing is required
- Food piece sizes designed to minimize choking risk
- Tongue force and control is required to move the food and keep it within the mouth for chewing and oral processing
- Tongue force is required to move the bolus for swallowing
- Pain or fatigue on chewing
- Missing teeth, or poorly fitting dentures

Although descriptions are provided, use IDDSI Testing methods to decide if the food meets IDDSI ▼ 6 Soft & Bite-Sized guidelines.

▼⑥ SOFT & BITE-SIZED TESTING METHODS

See also IDDSI Testing Methods document or
www.iddsi.org/framework/food-testing-methods/

Fork Pressure Test

- Pressure from a fork held on its side can be used to 'cut,' break apart or flake this texture into smaller pieces

- When a sample the size of a thumb nail (1.5 cm x 1.5 cm) is pressed with the tines of a fork to a pressure where the thumb nail blanches to white, the sample squashes, breaks apart, changes shape, and does not return to its original shape when the fork is removed.

Spoon Pressure Test

- Pressure from a spoon held on its side can be used to 'cut' or break this texture into smaller pieces.

- When a sample the size of a thumb nail (1.5 cm x 1.5 cm) is pressed with the base of a spoon, the sample squashes, breaks apart, changes shape, and does not return to its original shape when the spoon is removed.

Chopstick Test (where forks are not available)

- Chopsticks can be used to break this texture into smaller pieces or puncture food

Finger Test (where forks are not available)

- Use a sample the size of a thumb nail (1.5 cm x 1.5 cm). It is possible to squash a sample of this texture using finger pressure such that the thumb and index finger nails blanch to white. The sample breaks apart and will not return to its initial shape once pressure is released.

FOOD SPECIFIC, OR OTHER EXAMPLES

The following items may be suitable for IDDSI ▼⑥ Soft & Bite-Sized:

Meat

- Cooked, tender meat no bigger than
  - Pediatric: 8 mm pieces
  - Adults: 15 mm = 1.5 x 1.5 cm pieces

- If texture cannot be served soft and tender at 1.5 cm x 1.5 cm (as confirmed with fork/spoon pressure test), serve minced and moist

Fish

- Soft enough cooked fish to break into small pieces with fork, spoon or chopsticks no larger than:
  - Pediatric: 8 mm pieces
  - Adults: 15 mm = 1.5 cm pieces
- No bones or tough skins

Casserole/Stew/Curry

- Liquid portion (e.g. sauce) must be thick (as per clinician recommendations)
- Can contain meat, fish or vegetables if final cooked pieces are soft and tender and no larger than:
  - Pediatric: 8 mm pieces
  - Adults: 15 mm = 1.5 cm pieces
- No hard lumps

Fruit

- Serve minced or mashed if cannot be cut to soft & bite-sized pieces
  - Pediatric: 8 mm pieces
  - Adults: 15 mm = 1.5 cm pieces
- Fibrous parts of fruit are not suitable
- Drain excess juice
- Assess individual ability to manage fruit with high water content (e.g. watermelon) where juice separates from solid in the mouth during chewing

Vegetables

- Steamed or boiled vegetables with final cooked size of:
  - Pediatric: 8 mm pieces
  - Adults: 15 mm = 1.5 cm pieces
- Stir fried vegetables may be too firm and are not soft or tender. Check softness with fork/spoon pressure test

Cereal

- Smooth with soft, tender lumps no bigger than:
  - Pediatric: 8 mm pieces
  - Adults: 15 mm = 1.5 cm pieces
- Texture fully softened
- Any excess milk or liquid must be drained and/or thickened to appropriate thickness level

Bread

- No regular, dry bread, sandwiches or toast of any kind
- Use IDDSI Level 5 Minced & Moist sandwich recipe video (https://youtu.be/W7bOufqmz18)
- Pre-gelled 'soaked' breads that are very moist and gelled through the entire thickness

Rice, Couscous, Quinoa

- Not particulate/grainy, sticky, or glutinous

▼ SOFT & BITE-SIZED SOFTNESS TESTS

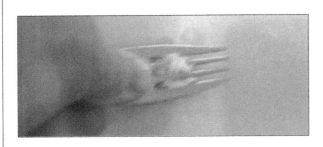

Thumbnail blanched white

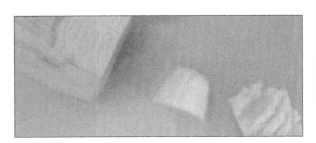

Sample squashes and does not return to its original shape when pressure is released

▼ SOFT & BITE-SIZED FOOD MUST PASS BOTH FOOD PIECE SIZE & SOFTNESS TESTS!

 For Children:
Food pieces no bigger than 8 mm x 8 mm lump size

 For Adults:
Food pieces no bigger than 1.5 cm x 1.5 cm lump size

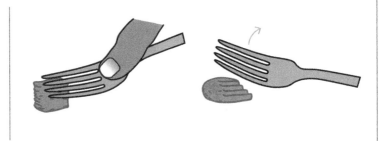

FOOD TEXTURES THAT POSE A CHOKING RISK

Examples are drawn from international autopsy reports.

- **Hard or dry textures are a choking risk because** they require good chewing ability to break down and mix with saliva to make them moist enough to be safe to swallow.
  - Examples of hard or dry textures: nuts, raw carrots, crackling, hard crusty rolls

- **Fibrous or tough textures are a choking risk because** they require good chewing ability, and sustained chewing ability to break down to small enough pieces that are safe to swallow.
  - Examples of fibrous or tough textures: steak, pineapple

- **Chewy textures are a choking risk because** they are sticky and can become stuck to the roof of the mouth, the teeth or cheeks and fall into the airway.
  - Examples of chewy textures: candies/lollipops/sweets, cheese chunks, marshmallows, chewing gum, sticky mashed potatoes

- **Crispy textures are a choking risk because** they require good chewing ability to break down and mix with saliva to make them soft, rounded and moist enough to be safe to swallow.
  - Examples of crispy textures: crackling, crisp bacon, some dry cereals

- **Crunchy textures are a choking risk because** they require good chewing ability, and sustained chewing ability to break them into small enough pieces and mix with saliva so that they are safe to swallow.
  - Examples of crunchy textures: raw carrots, raw apples, popcorn

- **Sharp or spiky textures are a choking risk because** they require good chewing ability to break them into small enough, soft, rounded pieces and moist enough to be safe to swallow.
  - Examples of sharp or spiky textures: dry corn chips

- **Crumbly textures are a choking risk because** they need good tongue control to bring crumbly pieces together and mix with enough saliva to hold together to be moist and safe to swallow.
  - Examples of crumbly textures: dry cakes, dry cookies, dry biscuits or scones

- **Seeds, pips and the white parts of fruit are a choking risk because** they are hard, and part of other hard, fibrous textures, making it a complex process to separate and remove them from the mouth.
  - Examples of seeds, pips and white parts of fruit: apple or pumpkin seeds, the white part of oranges

- **Skins, husks or outer shells are a choking risk because** the pieces are often fibrous, spiky, and dry needing good chewing skills to make the pieces smaller, and enough saliva to make it moist, OR enough skill to remove the pieces from the mouth. These small pieces become stuck to teeth and gums and catch in the throat when swallowed.
  - Examples of skins, husks or outer shells: pea shells, grape skin, bran, psyllium

- **Bone or gristle is a choking risk because** these pieces are hard and not usually chewed and swallowed. They require good tongue skills to remove them from the food texture they are attached to, and then remove the bone or gristle from the mouth.
  - Examples of bone or gristle: chicken bones, fish bones

- **Round, or long shaped foods are a choking risk because** if they are not chewed into small pieces and are swallowed whole, their shape can completely block the airway causing choking.
  - Examples of round or long shaped foods: sausages, grapes

- **Sticky or gummy textures are a choking risk because** they are sticky and can become stuck to the roof of the mouth, the teeth or cheeks and fall into the airway. They require sustained and good chewing ability to reduce stickiness by adding saliva to make them safe to swallow.
  - Examples of chewy textures: nut butter, overcooked oatmeal, edible gelatin, Konjac containing jelly, sticky rice cakes, candy

- **Stringy textures are a choking risk because** the string can be difficult to break and the flesh can become trapped with part in the mouth and part in the throat tied together by the stringy texture.
  - Examples of stringy textures: green string beans, rhubarb

- **Mixed thin-thick textures are a choking risk because** they require an ability to hold the solid piece in the mouth while the thin liquid portion is swallowed. After the liquid portion is swallowed, the solid pieces are chewed and swallowed. This is a very complex oral task.
  - Examples of mixed thin-thick textures: soup with food pieces, cereal pieces with milk, bubble tea

- **Complex food textures are a choking risk because** they require an ability to chew and manipulate a variety of food textures in one mouthful.
  - Examples of complex food textures: hamburgers, hot dogs, sandwiches, meatballs and spaghetti, pizza

- **Floppy textures are a choking risk because** if they are not chewed into small pieces they become thin and wet and can form a covering over the opening of the airway, stopping air from flowing.
  - Examples of floppy textures: lettuce, thinly sliced cucumbers, baby spinach leaves

- **Juicy food textures where the juice separates from the food when chewing are a choking risk because** they require the person to be able to swallow the juice while controlling the solid piece in the mouth. Once the juice has been swallowed, good chewing skills are needed to break the food into smaller pieces for safe swallowing. It is a complex oral task.
  - Examples of juicy food textures: watermelon

- **Hard skins or crusts formed during cooking or heating are a choking risk because** they require good chewing skills to break them down into smaller pieces while mixed with other food textures not affected by the heating process.

IDDSI Test Methods Document

In this appendix, we have reprinted information for IDDSI Testing Methods. For the most current information, consult www.iddsi.org/Testing-Methods

FOODS

Research to date in the area of food texture measurement requires complex and expensive machinery such as Food Texture Analyzers. Given the difficulty with access to such equipment and the expertise required for testing and interpretation, many existing national terminologies have used detailed descriptors to describe food texture instead.

The systematic review demonstrated that the properties of hardness, cohesiveness and slipperiness were important factors for consideration (Steele et al., 2015). In addition, size and shape of food samples have been identified as relevant factors for choking risk (Kennedy et al., 2014; Chapin et al., 2013; Japanese Food Safety Commission, 2010; Morley et al., 2004; Mu et al., 1991; Berzlanovich et al. 1999; Wolach et al., 1994; Centers for Disease Control and Prevention, 2002, Rimmell et al., 1995; Seidel et al., 2002).

In view of this information, measurement of foods needs to capture both the mechanical properties (e.g. hardness, cohesiveness, adhesiveness etc.) and the geometrical or shape attributes of the food. The IDDSI descriptions of food texture and characteristics, food texture requirements and restrictions have been generated from existing national terminologies and the literature describing properties that increase risk for choking.

IDDSI provides testing methods that use forks and spoons to minimize the need for subjectivity that often accompanies description-based methods. Forks and spoons were chosen as they are inexpensive, easily accessible and available in most food preparation and dining environments. A combination of tests may be required to determine which level a food fits into. Testing methods for purees, soft, firm and solid foods include: The Fork Drip test, Spoon Tilt Test, Fork or Spoon Pressure Test, Chopstick Test and Finger Test. Videos showing examples of these testing methods can be found at: www.iddsi.org/framework/food-testing-methods/

FORK DRIP TEST

Thick drinks and fluid foods (Levels 3 and 4) can be tested by assessing whether they flow through the tines/prongs of a fork and comparing against the detailed descriptions of each level. Fork Drip Rests are described in existing National terminologies in Australia, Ireland, New Zealand and the United Kingdom (Atherton et al., 2007; IASLT and Irish Nutrition & Dietetic Institute 2009; National Patient Safety Agency, Royal College Speech & Language Therapists, British Dietetic Association, National Nurses Nutrition Group, Hospital Caterers Association 2011).

Images for 3 Liquidised / 3 Moderately Thick are shown below.

Drips slowly or in dollops/strands through the tines/prongs of a fork.

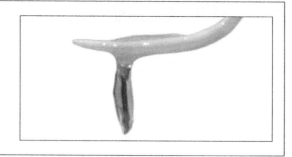

Images for 4 Pureed / 4 Extremely Thick are shown below.

- Sits in a mound or pile above the fork

- A small amount may flow through and form a short tail below the fork. Does not dollop, flow or drip continuously through the fork prongs.

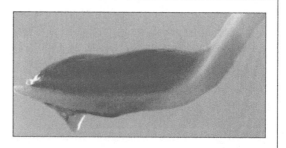

SPOON TILT TEST

The Spoon Tilt Test is used to determine the stickiness of the sample (adhesiveness) and the ability of the sample to hold together (cohesiveness). The Spoon Tilt Test is described in existing National terminologies in Australia, Ireland, New Zealand and the United Kingdom (Atherton et al., 2007; IASLT and Irish Nutrition & Dietetic Institute 2009; National Patient Safety Agency, Royal College Speech & Language Therapists, British Dietetic Association, National Nurses Nutrition Group, Hospital Caterers Association 2011).

The Spoon Tilt Test is used predominantly for measures of samples in Levels 4 and 5. The sample should:

- Be cohesive enough to hold its shape on the spoon

- A full spoonful must plop off the spoon, if the spoon is titled or turned sideways; a very gentle flick (using only fingers and wrist) may be necessary to dislodge the sample from the spoon, but the sample should slide off easily with very little food left on the spoon. A thin film remaining on the spoon after the Spoon Tilt Test is acceptable, however, you should still be able to see the spoon through the thin film; i.e. the sample should not be firm and sticky

- A scooped mound may spread or slump very slightly on a plate

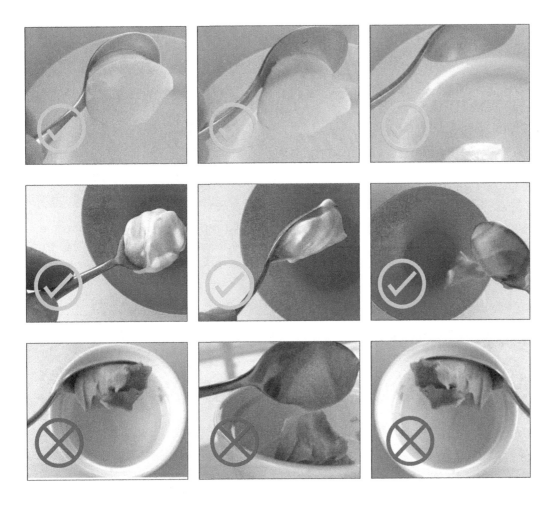

SOFT, FIRM AND HARD FOOD TEXTURE ASSESSMENT

For soft, hard or firm food, the fork has been chosen to assess food texture as it can uniquely be used for assessment of mechanical properties associated with hardness, in addition to assessment of shape attributes such as particle size.

ASSESSING FOR 4 MM PARTICLE SIZE COMPLIANCE

For adults, the average particle size of chewed solid foods before swallowing measures 2–4 mm (Peyron et al., 2004; Woda et al., 2010). The slots/gaps between the tines/prongs of a standard metal fork typically measure 4 mm, which provides a useful compliance measure for particle size of foods at ⑤ Minced & Moist. For determining particle size safety for infants, samples that are smaller than the maximum width of the child's fifth fingernail (littlest finger) should not cause a choking risk as this measurement is used to predict the internal diameter of an endotracheal tube in the pediatric population (Turkistani et al., 2009).

ASSESSING FOR 15 MM (1.5 CM) PARTICLE SIZE COMPLIANCE

For hard and soft solid foods, a maximum food sample size of 1.5 cm x 1.5 cm is recommended, which is the approximate size of the adult human thumb nail (Murdan, 2011). The entire width of a standard fork also measures approximately 1.5 cm as shown in the images below. 1.5 cm x 1.5 cm particle size is recommended for ⑥ Soft & Bite-sized to reduce risk associated with asphyxiation from choking on food (Berzlanovich et al., 2005; Bordsky et al., 1996; Litman et al., 2003).

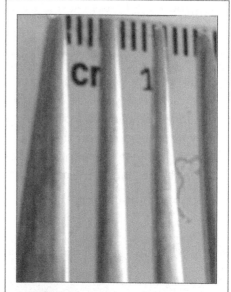

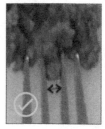 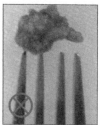

Compliance with 4 mm particle size can be demonstrated with a fork, as shown in the images.

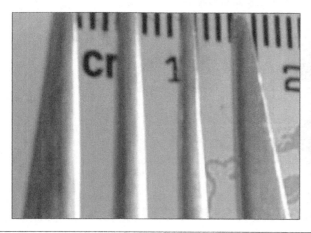 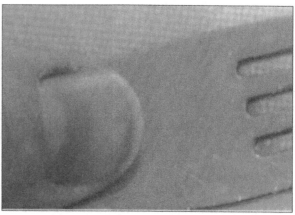

FORK PRESSURE TEST AND SPOON PRESSURE TEST

A fork can be applied to the food sample to observe its behaviour when pressure is applied. Pressure applied to the food sample has been quantified by assessment of the pressure needed to make the thumb nail blanch noticeably to white, as demonstrated by the arrows in the image at left.

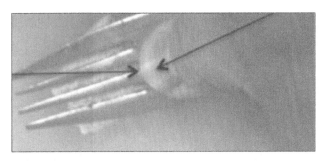

The pressure applied to make the thumb nail blanch has been measured at approximately 17 kPa. This pressure is consistent with tongue force used during swallowing (Steele et al., 2014). In the image at right, pressure is being demonstrated in kilopascals (kPa) using an Iowa Oral Performance Instrument. This is one device that can be used to measure tongue pressure.

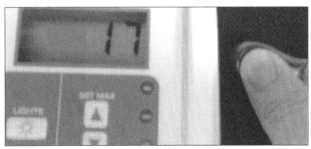

For assessment using the Fork Pressure Test, it is recommended that the fork be pressed onto the food sample by placing the thumb onto the bowl of the fork (just above the prongs) until blanching is observed, as shown in the image at right. It is appreciated that forks are not used/readily available in some parts of the world. Pressure applied using the base of a teaspoon may provide a useful alternative.

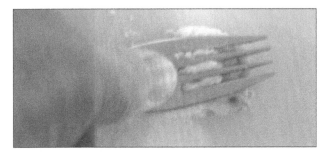

CHOPSTICK TEST AND FINGER TEST

Assessment with chopsticks has been included in the IDDSI test methods. Finger tests have been incorporated in recognition that this may be the most accessible method in some countries.

FORK/SPOON SEPARATION TEST

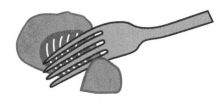

Must be able to break food apart easily with the side of a fork or spoon

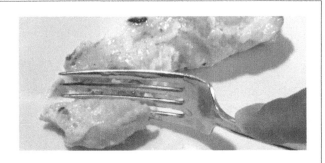

Made in the USA
Monee, IL
24 August 2023